Ethical Decision-Making
in Therapy Practice

Ethical Decision-Making in Therapy Practice

by
Julius Sim
BA MSc PhD MCSP

Professor, Department of Physiotherapy Studies,
Keele University, Keele, UK

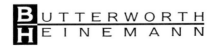
BUTTERWORTH
HEINEMANN

Butterworth-Heinemann
Linacre House, Jordan Hill, Oxford OX2 8DP
A division of Reed Educational and Professional Publishing Ltd

 A member of the Reed Elsevier plc group

OXFORD BOSTON JOHANNESBURG
MELBOURNE NEW DELHI SINGAPORE

First published 1997

British Library Cataloguing in Publication Data
A catalogue record for this book is available from the British Library

Library of Congress Cataloguing in Publication Data
A catalogue record for this book is available from the Library of Congress

ISBN 0 7506 2173 7

Composition by Scribe Design, Gillingham, Kent, UK
Printed and bound in Great Britain by Biddles Ltd, Guildford and Kings Lynn

Contents

Preface

This book has been written in recognition of a number of professional and theoretical developments in health care in general, and the therapies in particular. Above all, there has been a growing recognition in recent years of the need to subject clinical practice in the therapy professions to ethical scrutiny. It has become clear that the everyday work of therapists involves decisions and actions which have wide-ranging implications for the welfare, dignity and independence of their patients and clients. These are fundamentally moral issues. Additionally, as the therapies have gained greater clinical autonomy and higher professional status, there has been a concern to explore the conceptual and philosophical foundations of these professions – occupational therapy has perhaps led the way here. A key part of this movement is to analyse the moral basis of professional practice. Meanwhile, within health care in general there has been a call for a greater focus on 'philosophical medical ethics', involving the critical analysis of ethical issues, and correspondingly less emphasis on 'traditional medical ethics', which rely on the accepted, and somewhat unreflective, collective morality of individual professions, particularly as this is expressed in professional codes (Gillon, 1986). Factors such as these have brought ethics into prominence in professional thinking.

Just as the study of mental health requires an awareness of fundamental psychological concepts and mechanisms, and an understanding of pathology rests upon a grasp of basic principles of histology and physiology, so the study of ethics requires that certain fundamental concepts and principles of moral philosophy are understood. Accordingly, the first two chapters of this book are largely devoted to this topic. This reflects my belief that therapists must attempt to stand back from their instinctive or intuitive responses to ethical issues and subject them to critical analysis within a clear theoretical framework (which is not to say that these intuitive responses will not ultimately be found to be justified).

Owing to limitations of space, I have restricted the focus of the book to the ethics of clinical practice, and have not attempted to explore the important ethical issues that arise in therapy research. Similarly, although fundamental distinctions between ethics and the law are drawn in the opening chapter, no attempt is made within the remainder of the book to address legal issues. This is not only because of limited space, but also in recognition of the differences that exist in the law from country to country (and, in the USA, from state to state).

I have tried to concentrate on those areas of health care ethics which are likely to be of greatest relevance to therapists. Issues such as abortion and organ transplantation have not been addressed, even though they give rise to considerable ethical difficulties, and are by no means irrelevant to the work of some therapists. Where issues of concern to therapists have not been addressed, or have been considered only briefly, I hope that the coverage of fundamental concepts and principles within the book will provide readers with a sound basis on which to explore these specific issues for themselves.

Inevitably, a book on ethics will raise more questions than it will answer. Indeed, I have provided very few 'solutions' to the ethical conflicts that are identified in the chapters to follow. This reflects two important considerations: first, that a single 'correct' answer to an ethical conflict rarely exists; second, that an analytical approach to ethical decision-making requires that therapists should use basic concepts and principles to work through ethical problems in order to reach their own conclusions. A 'recipe book' approach is no more appropriate in ethical decision-making than it is in clinical decision-making.

Finally, I would like to express my gratitude to a number of people who have provided help or inspiration for this book. I would like to thank David McNaughton, who has greatly enlightened and clarified my thinking on moral philosophy with such patience and kindness. Similarly, I am very grateful to Ruth

Purtilo for stimulating discussions of many ethical issues within therapy practice, and for encouraging my work in this area over a number of years. I would also like to thank Sally French for helpful and constructive comments on the first draft of the manuscript. Lastly, Jackie Waterfield has not only provided numerous helpful comments on the content of the book, but also given me immense support and encouragement throughout its development.

The shortcomings of this book are, needless to say, my own responsibility, and the conclusions it reaches do not necessarily reflect the views of those whose help I have acknowledged above.

JS

1

Introduction to ethics

Recent years have seen an increasing interest in and concern for the ethical implications of medicine and health care. Much of this has no doubt been prompted by the technological advances that have been made in areas such as organ transplantation, genetic engineering, and life-support systems (Jennett, 1986; Lamb, 1990). In addition, natural phenomena such as the current AIDS pandemic have created dramatic ethical problems of their own. Meanwhile, there seems to have been an increasingly critical eye directed at hitherto sacrosanct institutions in society, notably the police, the judiciary, the church, and of course medicine. Whereas previously the activities and values of these professions and institutions enjoyed widespread public endorsement, there is now far more questioning of their role. Indeed, this has been carried to extremes in some areas, with militant animal rights activists taking drastic measures against vivisectionists and the food industry in the United Kingdom, and fundamentalist 'pro-life' groups threatening the lives of abortionists in the United States. Setting such extreme cases aside, there remains a general feeling that the values and preferences that control the delivery of health care should not be those of the professional alone (Williamson, 1992; Hopkins *et al.*, 1994; Rigge, 1994). Health care does not enjoy the same public and professional moral consensus that it perhaps did in the past.

This public concern with the morality of medicine and health care has been mirrored in the professions working in these areas. The nursing profession in particular has taken a great interest in the ethical implications of its practice. It is rare to find an issue of the *Journal of Advanced Nursing* that does not contain at least one paper on ethics, and a specialist journal, *Nursing Ethics*, has recently been launched. The therapy professions have shown a similar concern, though at present the body of literature on matters of ethics in areas such as occupational therapy and physiotherapy is limited.

Perhaps one reason for the comparative neglect of ethical issues in the literature of the therapy professions is that such issues are not so immediately apparent as those which arise in other areas of health care. In medicine and surgery, the ethical considerations underlying euthanasia, abortion, organ transplantation, and the like, are readily apparent, and command considerable public comment and debate. The ethical issues arising in the daily work of a speech and language therapist, in contrast, are less obvious. Rather than wrestling with issues of life and death, therapists are likely to have to deal with more apparently mundane ethical matters, for example:

- How should we determine treatment priorities within a caseload, especially under resource constraints?
- Are some patients more deserving of treatment than others, and if so on what grounds?
- Should we always obtain informed consent before treating a patient? If so, how 'informed' must this consent be, and what form should it take?
- To what extent is it permissible to 'persuade' patients or clients to pursue a course of action when they seem unwilling to do so?
- Is it justifiable to persevere with treatment that is proving ineffective, just because continued treatment has been recommended?
- Under what circumstances is it permissible to cause patients discomfort or pain?
- Can it be right to mislead patients as to their diagnoses, or the nature of the treatment they are being given?
- With whom is it permissible to discuss personal information about a patient or the details of his or her treatment?
- To what degree of personal risk should therapists be expected to expose themselves in the course of their work?
- What influence should third-party reimbursement have upon treatment prescription and continuation?

- What action should we take with respect to colleagues whom we regard as incompetent, or whose conduct we regard as unethical?

While the stakes are normally not so high in the therapy professions as they are in certain areas of medical practice, this does not mean that ethical issues are only of minor concern to therapists. As Melia has commented in respect of nursing:

> Moral dilemmas of the 'do or die' variety help us to focus upon the moral choices we must make, and so debating ethical dilemmas is a useful exercise. We should not, however, allow the big dilemmas to detract from the more routine moral choices involved in nursing. (Melia, 1989:1)

Indeed, the fact that these 'routine moral choices' are likely to be overlooked, whereas more life-and-death issues tend to draw themselves to our attention in a dramatic manner, suggests that we should pay particular heed to this first category. Moreover, whatever the 'public' prominence of certain issues, we need ultimately to consider what is of concern and significance to patients and clients themselves:

> As occupational therapists we face dilemmas in day-to-day practice that may not be as dramatic as those discussed in the media: however, to the individual patients and families involved they are crucial. (Hansen, 1988:279)

Edwards provides illustrations of the seemingly trivial transactions between practitioner and client which nonetheless are ethically significant:

> Consider actions such as moving a person from one chair to another without speaking to the client; removing the coat from a conscious, confused client without their permission; preventing a confused, elderly client from leaving a day hospital; coercing a person with learning difficulties into having a bath, or a wash; and so on. (Edwards, 1996:11)

In addressing the ethical issues that arise in clinical practice, therapists can learn much from the literature that exists on the ethics of medical practice. However, as Caplan (1988) indicates, the medical focus of this literature tends to embody certain assumptions about the nature of professional practice which limits its direct relevance to therapists. Among these assumptions are the following:

- The situations depicted are often based on curative interventions for acute conditions with a clear-cut diagnosis, whereas therapists are often involved in the management of chronic or progressive problems, the nature of which is sometimes unclear.
- The medical relationships portrayed are generally 'discrete, finite, and episodic' (Caplan, 1988:312), whereas contact between therapist and client tends to be long term, built around a series of clinical encounters.
- The relationships described are very often one to one, between a doctor and a patient. In contrast, the ethical problems faced by therapists commonly occur within the context of a multidisciplinary team.
- Similarly, within acute medical settings, the roles of the patient and the practitioner tend to be passive and active respectively, whereas in rehabilitation settings this model is replaced by one of mutual activity and cooperation, involving each party more or less equally (Scofield, 1993).
- As has already been noted, in traditional discussions of the ethics of medicine, the stakes are often very high, in terms of matters of life and death. In therapy, on the other hand, the issues are more commonly to do with such things as a client's long-term functional independence, experience of pain, or ability to communicate. This difference in scale tends to be reflected in a different weighting of various values, such that we cannot always transpose or, as it were, extrapolate ethical conclusions reached in the medical sphere to the field of therapy.

In a number of ways, then, a fresh and distinctive perspective needs to be taken upon the ethics of therapy practice.

The central role of ethics in health care

It might be asked why ethical considerations should be of special concern in health care. There are a number of reasons for this. In the first instance, health care practitioners generally see themselves as working as members of a profession. One of the key characteristics of such an occupational group is the presence of an ethical framework for professional practice (Sim, 1985).

Second, there are particular features of the relationship between therapist and patient or client which call for a special moral awareness. There is characteristically an imbalance of power and expertise in this relationship, with the patient occupying a relatively dependent role, even in cases where an apparently equal partnership exists between patient and practitioner. This creates a need to protect and/or promote the interests and dignity of patients (within certain limits) in circumstances in which they are unable to do so fully themselves. In addition, this relationship is typically characterized as a 'caring' one. The idea of caring is a fundamentally moral one (Noddings, 1984), and is often taken as a basis for the ethics of nursing (Brown *et al.*, 1992; Tschudin, 1992).

Perhaps the strongest argument for the moral basis of health care lies in the concept of health itself. There are many things, such as money, knowledge, fame and status, whose ultimate value we can dispute. However, health would seem to be self-evidently a good thing, as it is the precondition for almost everything else we value; as Seedhouse (1986) puts it, health is 'the foundations for achievement'. Good health is a valuable thing by definition, and is therefore something which we should seek to promote. Health care as an activity is hence a form of moral work:

> To speak of health is to refer to an essentially desirable state of affairs, while to speak of illness is to characterise a state of being as inherently undesirable. It follows from this that actions in the sphere of health care, in so far as they succeed or fail in improving the health of the patient, are either desirable or undesirable. As such, they can appropriately be evaluated in moral terms, such as 'right' and 'wrong'. (Sim, 1990:426)

This argument would seem to be particularly relevant to therapists' professional practice. The activities of physiotherapists, occupational therapists and speech and language therapists are closely tied to the functional capabilities of the individual, and it is the integrity of these functions that determines much of what the individual is able to achieve (though not necessarily *all* that the individual can achieve, as health embraces far more than functional capabilities).

This idea of health as a normative concept further suggests that ethical considerations are in a sense prior to more technical aspects of professional knowledge. It is only once it has been established that it is morally appropriate to intervene in the lives of others that we should consider the appropriate ways in which we should do so. To put it another way, ethics provides us with the proper *ends* of professional care, whereas technical knowledge and skills provide the *means*.

The professional accountability of the therapist

The notion of 'responsibility' or 'accountability' is a key issue in professional practice in health care (Baly, 1984; Sumerling, 1994). It is worth clarifying the different ways in which therapists may find themselves accountable. Adapting a typology proposed by Dimond (1995), three forms of accountability can be identified: legal, ethical and professional. These are displayed diagrammatically in Table 1.1.

While these spheres of accountability overlap to a certain degree, in other ways they are distinct from one another. The

Table 1.1 Sources of ethical, legal and professional accountability

Legal accountability	Ethical accountability	Professional accountability
Requirements of the Criminal Law	Responsibilities to patients and clients	Responsibilities to the good name of the profession, in general terms
Requirements of the Civil Law: - the law of contract - the law of tort	Responsibilities to patients' and clients' families and carers	Specific responsibilities to the professional body (e.g. COT, APTA, CSLT)
Other statutory demands: - Health and Safety legislation - Employment law	Responsibilities to society in general Responsibilities to professional colleagues	Specific responsibilities to the statutory body (e.g. the CPSM in the UK, state and federal authorities and licensure bodies in the USA)

precise relationship between the legal and ethical demands of accountability can be problematic, and is worth examining in some detail.

Ethics and the law

Many of the areas on which there is ethical controversy are also of legal concern. Indeed, the moral debate is often triggered by some form of legal action; for example, in the USA, the cases of Karen Quinlan and Nancy Cruzan (euthanasia), and in the UK, the Gillick case (teenage contraception), the Arthur case (euthanasia) and the Bolam case (informed consent). Therapists often have to be responsive to, and work within the confines of, specific pieces of legislation, e.g. the Americans with Disabilities Act (1990) and the Patient Self-Determination Act (1991) in the USA, and the Children Act (1989) and the Access to Health Records Act (1990) in the UK. In addition, therapists are governed by legislation specifically covering their professional activity. There are various licensure laws through the various states in the USA, and in the UK speech and language therapists are subject to the NHS (Speech Therapists) Regulations (1974), while occupational therapists and physiotherapists are governed by the Professions Supplementary to Medicine Act (1960).

It is important, however, to appreciate the differences between the law and morality, not only because the two are often confused during the course of discussion of controversial issues, but also because an understanding of each discipline depends upon a clear grasp of its role and scope. The demands which morality and the law make, and the purposes which they each serve, should be distinguished in a number of respects:

- The law tends to specify the minimum of what you should or should not do. It sets a standard of conduct below which you must not fall. In contrast, morality encourages you not just to attain a certain standard, but in many cases to go beyond it; to strive to lead an even better life. There's always that bit more you can do to be a morally better person, or to show more consideration for others, but as long as you keep within the specific demands of the law, that is more or less the end of the matter. Accordingly, the law is primarily concerned with imposing prohibitions (i.e. that which we must not do), whereas morality is concerned not only with prohibitions but also with prescriptions (i.e. that which we must do).

- The law does not necessarily cover all the aspects of life which it potentially could – there tends to be a certain threshold below which the law doesn't apply (this is known as the principle of *de minimis non curat lex*, 'the law does not concern itself with trivial matters'). This is not so much the case with ethics. As we have noted, although special concern must be given to issues, such as abortion or euthanasia, which involve life-and-death choices, matters which may seem trivial in comparison are nonetheless worthy of serious ethical scrutiny.

- Closely linked to the previous point is the fact that the law can be changed at any time by human action. Something which was legal on Tuesday may, with a change in the law, become illegal on Wednesday. However, except perhaps in some systems of religious morality, something cannot just be decreed good or bad or right or wrong and automatically become so. Changes in morality certainly do occur, but more by a process of evolution. Essentially, morality may *alter*, but the law can be *altered*.

- The law has to arrive at a single determinate conclusion on a given case (though not everybody will necessarily agree that it is the right one). This may be in terms of a verdict of 'guilty' or 'not guilty' in a criminal case, or a monetary sum for compensation in a civil case. The law seeks to make unambiguous judgments on the basis of factual evidence, and once it has done so the matter tends to be more or less closed. Ethics, on the other hand, can accommodate ambiguity and the absence of a specific conclusion. Very few matters are settled once and for all in ethics – it is always an 'open question', and precedent, in the form of a previous decision, does not carry the same authority as it does in the law.

   However, in practical affairs such as health care ethics, there is always a need to decide on one course of action or another, otherwise one would be paralysed by indecision.

The point is, however, that you do not assume with certainty that the decision that is made on the particular occasion is the final word on the matter.
- Laws cannot conflict, or if they do so on rare occasions, this is seen as a defect in the law. Moral conflicts do occur, and when they do arise we do not necessarily see them as a defect in morality itself. Indeed, if there were no conflict between rights, duties, principles, etc., it is likely that we would have no need to engage in any form of ethical decision-making.

Important as the above distinctions are, perhaps the most crucial difference between morality and the law lies in the fact that not everything that is illegal is immoral, and vice versa. In the United Kingdom, it is illegal to sound the horn in a stationary vehicle, to smoke cannabis, to purchase alcohol outside certain prescribed hours – but for many people these are not necessarily immoral actions. Conversely, while many would feel that it is immoral to break a promise, embarrass or ridicule somebody in public, borrow something without permission, or to commit suicide, none of these are illegal in normal circumstances.

Figure 1.1 illustrates the relationship between ethics and the law, and indicates the way in which the overlap between the two is only partial. It also portrays another set of demands that may govern action – notions of prudence. Sometimes people follow a certain course of action not because the law requires them to, or because they feel morally impelled to do so, but because it is a

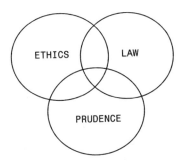

Figure 1.1 The relationship between ethical, legal and prudential considerations

wise or prudent course in terms of their own interests – they may simply wish to 'cover themselves'. To take a mundane example, there is no particular legal or moral necessity to insure your car against theft, but it is perhaps a very wise step to take. Equally, some actions are supported by considerations of all three types:

> Simon Rust is assessing a patient who has been referred to physiotherapy with acute neck pain. On the basis of the clinical findings, he has decided to perform a high velocity thrust manipulation to the appropriate level of the patient's vertebral column. However, before carrying out the technique, he explains the nature and purpose of the manipulation, and its possible side effects, to the patient, and asks for her consent to proceed.

Here, there are both legal and ethical reasons for obtaining a patient's consent to treatment – not to do so would deny freedom of choice to the patient, and proceeding with the technique without consent could constitute the tort of trespass to the person. In addition, it is prudent to seek consent in this situation, as doing so will serve to protect the therapist from adverse consequences. However, while all three reasons may support the same course of action, the legal and ethical motives are primarily related to the interests of the patient, whereas the prudential reasons are concerned with the therapist's interests. Particularly difficult situations can arise in which health professionals may have to sacrifice a concern for their own interests in order to pursue what they see as the morally required course of action; e.g. a therapist who feels impelled to 'blow the whistle' on dangerous or incompetent practices in a hospital may put his or her own career at risk.

What Figure 1.1 does not tell us is whether the demands of morality or those of the law should be paramount. However, from what has already been said on the relationship between the two, it seems clear that morality is (or should be) the basis for law, whereas it makes little sense to say that law is the basis for morality. As Downie and Calman (1994:42) point out, 'morality remains undetermined by law and can act as a critique of the law'. Morality, therefore, is the more fundamental set of imperatives, to which the law should be subject. Indeed, it is sometimes said that there is not necessarily a moral obligation to observe the law if it can be argued that the law in question is unjust.

Consider the following case, summarized from Bailey and Schwartzberg (1995):

> Gary Bernstein, an occupational therapist, has been treating Mrs Jaycynski for eight weeks following a stroke. At present, Mrs Jaycynski's progress seems to have reached a plateau. Nonetheless, Gary is a very experienced neurological therapist, and is convinced there is further improvement available. The insurance company funding the treatment operates a policy whereby, if no progress is shown at the end of each week, therapy will no longer be funded, and cannot be restarted. Gary feels inclined to falsify the treatment record in order to show an apparent improvement for this week, even though this is not the case, in order to secure further rehabilitation for Mrs Jaycynski.

Here, different spheres of accountability pull in different directions. The law, and no doubt institutional policy within the rehabilitation unit as well, would require that all treatment records are filled in accurately and honestly. However, from the ethical point of view, Gary might feel that although there is a moral requirement to maintain truthful records, this is outweighed in such a situation by the moral requirement to promote the client's welfare – on balance, the latter is seen by Gary to be his moral duty overall. Thus, Gary might decide to fulfil his perceived moral obligation at the cost of performing an action that contravenes institutional policy and the law.

'Ethical' and 'moral'

Before concluding this first chapter, it is important briefly to discuss the adjectives 'ethical' and 'moral', which have hitherto been used more or less interchangeably. These two terms can be used either descriptively or evaluatively. If we say that 'euthanasia is an ethical issue' or that there are 'moral dimensions to the question of treatment allocation', we are speaking in a descriptive way; we are simply saying that these topics can fall within the purview of ethical or moral deliberation. We are not, however, speaking evaluatively, because thus far we are not taking any particular moral stance on the questions of euthanasia or resource allocation. In this sense, there is no real difference between the terms 'ethical' and 'moral'.

If, on the other hand, we say that somebody is very 'moral' (or 'immoral'), or that a certain action was 'ethical' (or 'unethical'), we are making a value judgement, and in this usage the two terms carry a slightly different meaning. Thus, there is a general tendency to say that something is immoral if it goes against morality in a general sense, but that something is unethical if it goes against a specific code of moral behaviour associated with a particular professional role. It might be said that it is immoral for anybody to commit adultery, but that it is unethical (as well as immoral) for therapists to commit adultery with their patients.

Similarly, if we talk about a set of 'morals', we usually mean the standards by which an individual leads his or her life, whereas we refer to the 'ethics' of a professional collectivity, as in a 'code of professional ethics'. The term 'ethics' also refers, of course, to the theory of morality, otherwise known as 'moral philosophy'. The branch of ethics that has to do with making ethical decisions in concrete, real-life situations, and which is the primary focus of this book, is sometimes known as 'practical ethics', or 'applied ethics'.

Finally, a distinction should be made between ethics and etiquette. The notion of professional etiquette has to do with professional decorum and courtesy, and acceptable forms of interprofessional conduct. It has been suggested that many of the early codes of ethics in medicine were primarily concerned with such matters:

> A major portion of the issues addressed in such codes of etiquette were not moral issues in an immediate and strict sense, but rather questions of fees, advertisement, and the relation of physicians with non-orthodox practitioners. Such rules are not trivial. Codes of etiquette formally describe an important dimension of the mores of a group or profession. (Engelhardt, 1986:23)

Now, however, the notion of 'professional ethics' is generally seen to embrace wider concerns:

> Although everyone can applaud the desirability of showing respect to one's professional colleagues, such suggestions as promising never to question a physician's judgment sound oddly foreign within today's health care context. (Purtilo, 1989:36)

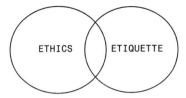

Figure 1.2 The relationship between ethics and etiquette

While, as Engelhardt points out, issues of professional etiquette are not necessarily trivial, they do not in most cases raise significant ethical issues. However, on some occasions a failure to observe accepted channels of communication, or a refusal to follow usual systems of patient referral, can have important implications for the welfare of the patient (Campbell *et al.*, 1992). Equally, moral considerations may on occasions require that rules of etiquette are disregarded – such as when these rules protect professional self-interest to the detriment of patient welfare (Sugarman, 1994). In both such situations, professional etiquette has moral significance.

Nonetheless, in most cases matters of etiquette do not require the sort of critical reflection involved in genuinely moral issues: 'You may be instructed by etiquette. Ethics demands you make judgments for yourself' (Fletcher *et al.*, 1995:5). It would seem, therefore, that the appropriate relationship between ethics and etiquette is that portrayed in Figure 1.2; while the two may sometimes overlap, on many occasions they are distinct from each other.

Conclusion

This chapter has attempted to examine some of the basic ideas underlying a concern for ethics in the therapy professions, and has suggested that therapists cannot rely totally on the ideas which have been generated within the ethics of medicine. This is not because therapists in some way have their 'own' ethics, but simply reflects the fact that the particular nature of professional practice in the therapies may demand an approach to ethical decision-making that is tailored to the kinds of activity and the sorts of client that are encountered in this area of health care.

An attempt has also been made to clarify some of the basic terminology within ethics. This task is as yet incomplete, and the following chapter will explore further the theoretical framework that is necessary for a critical analysis of specific ethical issues.

2

Ethical decision-making

This chapter will explore further the conceptual basis of ethical decision-making by examining the main ethical principles that are commonly used as a basis for ethical analysis. The notions of duties, rights and moral conflict will also be examined, and the chapter will conclude with a discussion of three approaches to ethical decision-making.

Ethical principles

The predominant approach to ethical decision-making in Western ethics is based on the idea that there are certain basic ethical principles. An ethical principle can be regarded as the statement of a fundamental ethical value or belief, which grounds and justifies specific ethical decisions and actions. Five such principles are commonly referred to. These primary principles will be discussed below, and the way in which secondary ethical principles can be derived from them will then be illustrated. The second half of this chapter will explore differing approaches to ethical decision-making.

Beneficence and non-maleficence

It is useful to consider these two principles together. The principle of beneficence states that one should strive to promote the interests of others by conferring benefits upon them. This may take one of two forms. One may either act to produce positive good for a person, or one may act in such a way as to remove a person from harm. Thus, to give food and water to a person, or perform some similar action which will give pleasure or satisfaction, is a beneficent act of the first sort. To throw a lifebelt to somebody in trouble in a swimming pool is an example of the second sort. Both have in common, however, that the individual is better off than previously as a result of one's action.

The principle of non-maleficence is not regarded as being a separate principle from beneficence by some writers (e.g. Frankena, 1963; Englehardt, 1986). However, it does seem to be saying something rather different: it states that one should seek to avoid inflicting harm on others. Whereas beneficence imposes a *positive* requirement on us to take certain steps to cause another person to be better off, non-maleficence requires us to *refrain* from doing that which would make another person worse off; it is a *negative* requirement.

Non-maleficence has tended to take pride of place within health care ethics. There is a famous medical maxim *primum non nocere* ('above all, do no harm'), thought to derive from the time of Hippocrates, which reflects the strong prohibition in health care against causing harm. Indeed, non-maleficence is often thought to be more pressing as a moral requirement than beneficence. There seem to be a number of reasons for this. First, failing to improve somebody's situation seems to be somehow less reprehensible than actually making somebody's situation worse. It is as if we bear an additional responsibility for an unfavourable outcome that we *caused* to happen, as opposed to one which we simply *allowed* to occur. Second, the sort of motives which are likely to prompt acts of maleficence are normally worse than those associated with failures to be beneficent; if we fail to help somebody in need, this is often due to insensitivity or indifference on our part, whereas if we harm somebody, this often represents a vindictive and malicious disposition.

Third, consistently observing the principle of non-maleficence is less onerous than in the case of beneficence. There are relatively few occasions on which we are likely to harm somebody through our actions, and it is reasonable, therefore, that we should always refrain from doing so. In contrast, the opportunity to do good for others is almost constantly present, and many would argue that it is not reasonable to expect us to be doing good for others at every moment, to the exclusion of all else (Sikora, 1993).

Similarly, while we do not necessarily recognize a duty to benefit each and every one of our fellow citizens, we do perhaps recognize a duty not to harm each and every one of them (Gillon, 1994a). On this basis, some regard non-maleficence as a *perfect* duty (i.e. one which must be fulfilled on every relevant occasion) and beneficence as an *imperfect* duty (i.e. one which must be fulfilled on some, but not all, relevant occasions).

Finally, it can be argued that a failure to observe the principle of non-maleficence has potentially far graver consequences for society than a corresponding neglect of beneficence. If we fail to do good for others, existence will certainly lose much of its essential humanity, and will lack the reciprocity that characterizes living in a community. However, life will probably still proceed at a minimally tolerable level; nobody will perform acts of kindness or offer assistance to others, but nor will people wilfully deceive, assault, injure or otherwise harm one another. In contrast, if we do not consistently forbear from performing maleficent acts, there is effectively no lower limit to the resulting deterioration in the quality of our existence.

In short, non-maleficence seems to be more indispensable to tolerable social life than beneficence. However, to say that nonmaleficence is *in general* a more urgent moral demand than beneficence is not to say that it will take priority in every individual situation. The particular circumstances of a case may dictate that the conferring of benefits is more important than the avoidance of harm. Furthermore, to maintain that non-maleficence is in some sense paramount – that it matters above all else – does not mean that it is *all* that matters. An approach to ethics that was only concerned to avoid harming other people, with little attention to the positive demands of morality, would be a rather minimalist one.

Respect for autonomy

Autonomy may be defined as the 'capacity to think, decide and act on the basis of such thought and decision freely and independently' (Gillon, 1986:60). The autonomous person determines for him- or herself what sort of life to lead, while the heteronomous person is one whose life is in the control of other people, external factors, or an internal factor which is somehow contrary to the person's 'true' wishes, such as weakness of will.

Autonomy is an aspect of liberty, but is a wider notion. Dworkin (1988:14) defines liberty as 'the ability of a person to do what she wants, to have (significant) options that are not closed or made less eligible by the actions of other agents'. If we physically constrain people, by imprisonment or involuntary admission to a mental hospital, we remove their liberty and an essential part of their autonomy, as previously defined. However, if we give false information, this does little to restrict the liberty of those whom we deceive – they can still come and go as they please, and can physically do more or less what they want – but it does impair their autonomy. Lacking this essential information, they can no longer act on the basis of rational decision-making. Hence, we can undermine a person's autonomy not only by restricting their freedom of action, but also by interfering with the factual and rational basis of such action.

Thus, there is both autonomy related to action and autonomy related to thought and decision-making. It is important to realize that a person may have lost autonomy of action, such as through severe physical impairment, while retaining autonomy of will and of thought. We must, therefore, be very wary of regarding such a person as non-autonomous overall (Gillon, 1986).

Having defined the concept of autonomy, the ethical principle of respect for autonomy can be seen as the requirement that we should protect the autonomy or self-determination of others. Indeed, it may also be seen to require us to go further than this and *enhance* their self-determination. The principle of respect for autonomy is in many ways central to health care in general, and to the activities of therapists in particular. If we return to Seedhouse's definition of health, which was touched upon in the previous chapter, it is clear that this is largely based on the idea of autonomy:

> A person's optimum state of health is equivalent to the state of the set of conditions which fulfil or enable a person to work to fulfil his or her realistic chosen and biological potentials. Some of these conditions are of the highest importance for all people. Others are variable dependent upon individual abilities and circumstances. (Seedhouse, 1986:61)

▲ Seedhouse stresses that individuals should choose their own potentials, and health professionals should not try to influence this choice, unless it undermines the individual's own central conditions for health or in some way interferes with the potentials of others. Thus, health care is fundamentally and inescapably concerned with the protection and promotion of autonomy.

If we turn to the professional role of the therapist, this argument appears in even sharper focus. At a fairly simple level, terms like 'functional capacity' or 'independent living' have clear affinities with the concept of autonomy, and basic physical functions such as locomotion and communication are preconditions for most higher-order achievements. More fundamentally, the notion of 'occupation', which lies at the heart of many models of occupational therapy, seems to be constructed around a model of the autonomous person:

> Occupational therapy provides service programs to assist individuals in meeting their human needs through the performance of those occupations (self-maintenance, productivity, leisure) that will lead to a satisfying and productive life. The major purpose is to develop and maintain the individual's capacity, throughout the life cycle, to perform with satisfaction to self and others those occupational tasks and roles essential to productive living and the mastery of self and the environment. (Reed and Sanderson, 1992:10)

Accordingly, freedom and autonomy have been identified by the American Occupational Therapy Association as a core value of occupational therapy (AOTA, 1993).

In some areas, the therapist's role may extend beyond the maintenance or restoration of autonomy to its creation or enhancement, for example in health promotion:

▲ In health promotion work, this is often called empowerment. It may involve information to enable clients to make choices or developing the clients' skills in analysing situations and making decisions through increased self-awareness and assertiveness. (Naidoo and Wills, 1994:109)

The autonomy we are concerned with at this juncture is that of the individual client or patient. We also hear talk of the concept of 'professional autonomy' (Øvretveit, 1985), the ability of a profession to control and regulate its own professional activities in an independent manner. The two sorts of autonomy should not be confused because, in each case, a very different set of interests is at stake, with distinct ethical implications (we will see in Chapter 9 that tension may exist between client autonomy and professional autonomy).

Respect for autonomy is therefore a crucial factor in many areas of health care ethics, and is particularly relevant to the concept of informed consent, to be examined in Chapter 3.

Respect for persons

The principle of respect for persons demands that we should deal with others with due consideration for their dignity as individuals, and that we should value the 'inherent worth and uniqueness of each person' (AOTA, 1993:1086). The tendency towards anonymity and 'depersonalization' that exists in health care settings lends considerable importance to this principle. It is grounded in ideas such as these:

🌿 Respecting the patient as person calls upon us to regard patients as unique individuals and to see them in the totality of their being, with physical, psychological, social, and spiritual dimensions alike....it is as persons that we are all fellow human beings, fellow members of the human community. (Corr and Corr, 1986:23)

A key element in this principle is Immanuel Kant's prohibition against using people merely as means (Paton, 1958). If one uses individuals simply as a means to one's own ends, without at the same time treating them as ends in themselves, such as in the course of experimentation, this is to fail to respect their essential human dignity.

It should be pointed out that many commentators do not recognize respect for persons as an independent principle (e.g. Gillon, 1994b; Beauchamp and Childress, 1994), and appear to identify it with the principle of respect for autonomy. There is indeed great similarity between the two, as autonomy is central to the notion of personhood: 'to impair a person's abilities to formulate and carry out aims and policies of his own devising is to that extent to destroy him as a person' (Downie and Telfer, 1969:20-1).

Nonetheless, there are a number of situations which would seem to be more usefully analysed in terms of respect for persons than in terms of autonomy. Moreover, there can be a tendency for the individuality of the person to get lost in discussions of general ethical principles, and the idea of individual dignity that underlies the principle of respect for persons helps in some small measure to counteract this.

Justice

Broadly speaking, the principle of justice requires that we should deal with others in a way that is fair and in accordance with their individual merit, and that we should 'act on the basis of a fair adjudication between competing claims' (Gillon, 1994b:185). More specifically, it insists that benefits and burdens within society should be apportioned in a way that is morally justifiable. For the ancient Greek philosopher Aristotle, this meant that everybody should be treated in the same way unless there are relevant differences between individuals which justify their being treated differently. Thus, justice goes further than a simple statement of equality ('treat everybody the same') to an acceptance that some inequalities may be justified in terms of the different needs and merits of individuals (Campbell, 1988).

There are two main varieties of justice. *Retributive justice* has to do with rewards and punishments, and is therefore of special relevance to areas such as the criminal law. Despite its name, it is not concerned solely with the idea of retribution; it also has to do with issues of restitution or compensation. The other variety of justice is *distributive justice*. This concerns the allocation of societal costs and benefits, and may take either a comparative or a non-comparative form. Non-comparative justice is where an individual receives what he or she needs and/or deserves. Comparative justice, on the other hand, has to do with the benefits received by one person relative to those received by others in society. Distributive justice will be a key issue when considering the management of health care resources in Chapter 7. Table 2.1 summarizes the five general principles that have been considered.

Table 2.1 Summary of basic ethical principles

Principle	Description	Key features
Beneficence	The positive requirement to promote the interests and well-being of others	Includes actions that will protect a person from harm, as well as those that will directly confer benefit. Illustrative issues – benevolent deception (Chapter 3), surrogate decision-making (Chapter 4), non-voluntary euthanasia (Chapter 6).
Non-maleficence	The negative requirement not to harm others	Often thought to be more stringent than beneficence. Illustrative issues – confidentiality (Chapter 5), voluntary and non-voluntary euthanasia (Chapter 6).
Respect for autonomy	The requirement to respect the self-determination of others	Usually only covers persons who are, or have previously been, autonomous. May require the enhancement, as well as the preservation, of a person's self-determination. Illustrative issues – truthfulness (Chapter 3), informed consent (Chapter 4), voluntary euthanasia (Chapter 6), advocacy (Chapter 9), suicide (Chapter 9).
Respect for persons	The requirement to respect the dignity and individuality of others	Closely linked with the principle of respect for autonomy, but covers both autonomous and non-autonomous persons. Requires that we should not use people as a means to an end. Illustrative issues – truthfulness (Chapter 3), privacy (Chapter 5), resource allocation (Chapter 7).
Justice	The requirement to treat others fairly	Can be analysed in terms of distributive and retributive justice. Differential treatment of others must be morally justifiable. Illustrative issues – resource allocation (Chapter 7), care of older people (Chapter 9).

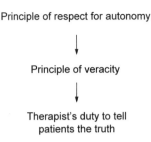

Figure 2.1 The relationship between a general principle, a secondary principle and a specific duty

Secondary principles

The five principles described above are, as they stand, rather abstract, and may not seem to have a direct connection with everyday ethical matters. However, on further examination it becomes clear that secondary principles can be derived from these general principles. These secondary principles are more focused, and generate specific duties in specific circumstances. Thus, the principle of respect for autonomy gives rise to the secondary principle of veracity, which in turn imposes a duty to convey truthful information to patients (see Figure 2.1).

As we will see when discussing specific issues, a number of such secondary principles can be derived from a single general principle, and equally a given secondary principle may be traced back to more than one general principle. Secondary principles begin to give us specific guidance in particular situations, which general principles cannot to the same degree. Conversely, general principles provide an indication as to why these secondary principles are important. We will return to this idea when discussing the justification of ethical decisions later in this chapter.

Moral rights and duties

Discussions of ethical issues are frequently framed in terms of rights and duties. It is worth briefly examining these two terms. A duty is essentially a moral requirement to do, or to refrain from doing, something. Duties can be derived from an ethical principle, as in the case of truth-telling just considered. Alternatively, they can be generated from specific actions of oneself or others, in which case they are generally referred to as obligations. Thus, if I make a promise to you, or do something to harm you, I am thereby under an obligation to keep the promise, or to make amends for the harm I have done you. Similarly, if you do a service for me, I am thereby under an obligation of gratitude to you.

Those duties or obligations which require one to do something are referred to as *positive* duties, while those which require one not to do something are known as *negative* duties. Some duties are general, and apply essentially to everybody, while others are special, and exist only in certain specific relationships, such as that between therapist and client. In all cases, a duty or obligation must be based on something more basic. One does not just have a duty; one has a duty *because of* a more fundamental ethical value, a past action, a special relationship, etc.

In contrast to a duty, a moral right can be defined as a morally justified claim. This does not mean that a right has to be claimed in order to be a right. Young children, comatose patients, or fetuses are commonly seen as possessing certain rights, even though they are in no position to claim them. A right is something to which we *have* a claim, i.e. an entitlement, not necessarily something to which we need *make* a claim (Sim, 1995). Such an entitlement may be to do something (e.g. the right to 'free speech'), in which case it is known as a right of action, or it may be an entitlement to receive something (e.g. the right to health care), when it is referred to as a right of recipience (Raphael, 1967).

If one has a right to do something, one thereby has a right not to do it. You cannot, therefore, have both a right and a duty to do something. However, it is generally the case that if you have a right, *someone else* has a corresponding duty. So, if a patient has a right to health care, someone else has a duty to provide it. Similarly, if we each have a right to free speech, others have a duty not to interfere with the expression of our views (provided that our exercise of this right does not infringe the rights of others).

Like duties, rights must be justified; they must be grounded in something more fundamental which gives them their moral authority. Too often, rights are claimed without any clear statement as to what justifies their status. As Harris (1985:xvi) points out, rights should feature in the *conclusion* of a moral argument, not in its *premises*.

Moral conflict

On occasions, more than one principle is at stake in a particular situation, and each of these principles may make conflicting demands. We will encounter specific examples in subsequent chapters, but it may be worth providing a brief illustration at this point:

> A 25-year-old unmarried man has severe vascular disease and it is recommended that his left foot be amputated to below the knee. He is advised that if he refuses to agree to this operation his chances of survival are very remote. He is adamant that he would rather die than be one-legged. He is strongly counselled and his family all advise him to have the operation. The ward sister arranges for a patient of similar age, who had the operation several years ago and who has since completed the marathon and adjusted very well to the amputation, to visit the patient and he shows him how he is enjoying life. The patient is not persuaded and still refuses to sign the consent form. Legal advice is taken that in the absence of any mental disorder he cannot be compelled to undergo the operation. A psychiatrist who visits him concludes that the patient is not mentally disordered and has decided on rational grounds that he would prefer death to an amputation. (Dimond, 1995:98–9)

There is a clear tension here between the principle of beneficence, which dictates that health professionals should strive to improve the patient's welfare, and the principle of respect for autonomy, which requires that the individual's wishes should be respected. This raises an important point about moral principles, which is that they are prima facie (i.e. provisional) rather than absolute (Ross, 1930). That is, a moral principle will dictate a certain course of action unless it conflicts with another moral principle, in which case some way must be found of deciding which of these principles should take precedence. If moral principles were regarded as absolute, on the other hand, a situation such as the one above could not be resolved, as by definition neither principle could yield to the other. As has already been suggested, we should be wary of assuming that one particular principle (e.g. non-maleficence) is intrinsically weightier than another (e.g. beneficence) when seeking to resolve a moral conflict. To do so is to take an unduly simplistic and mechanical approach to the issue. Although, within certain moral perspectives, some principles may well have a tendency to be more insistent than others, the facts of the specific situation at hand may not always support this assumption.

Sometimes a moral conflict can take a particularly acute form, known as a moral dilemma. Here, an individual has no choice but to perform one of two (or more) actions, each of which has morally undesirable consequences, and there seems to be no satisfactory way of assigning moral priority to one course of action over the other(s). A classic example of a moral dilemma occurs in the novel *Sophie's Choice* (Styron, 1980), in which a mother is given the choice of (a) selecting one of her two children to be saved, in which case the other child will be killed, or (b) making no such selection, thereby causing both children to die. On the one hand, favouring one child over the other in such circumstances seems to be a morally unacceptable choice, yet it also seems to be wrong not to save one of the children when given the opportunity to do so.

Three approaches to ethical decision-making

Having examined some of the key concepts within ethics, it is necessary to consider the actual process whereby ethical decisions are reached. Broadly speaking, there are three theoretical approaches that can be taken to the process of ethical decision-making: deontology, consequentialism and virtue ethics. These will be considered in turn.

Deontology

The deontological approach is firmly based on the general principles described in the previous section. Somebody who follows this approach would use these principles as the final test of a moral conflict. The deciding factor is whether the proposed course of action is in keeping with respect for autonomy, beneficence, etc. If it accords with one such prima facie principle but conflicts with another, an attempt will be made to determine which principle is the weightier in the circumstances. Thus, an occupational therapist working within a deontological framework would wish to ensure that all clients are fully informed and consulted as to the nature of their treatment or rehabilitation, in keeping with the principle of respect for autonomy. Equally, a physiotherapist would decline to inflict unpleasant or painful treatment on a seriously ill patient, so as not to infringe the principle of non-maleficence. As was noted above, the situation will sooner or later arise where two or more principles come into some degree of conflict, and some means of prioritizing among them will be required. Thus, in the second example above, it might be felt that it is justifiable to cause the patient discomfort because this is ultimately to the individual's benefit (i.e. fulfils the principle of beneficence), and that because this benefit is likely to be enduring, while the discomfort is perhaps only transitory, considerations of non-maleficence are outweighed in this instance by those of beneficence. A similar case might be made for the use of aversive techniques for self-injurious behaviour among clients with learning disabilities (Turnbull *et al.*, 1986).

Deontology recognizes that certain relationships, such as that between therapist and patient, may bring special duties with them, and may accordingly give special weight to these duties. The therapist may therefore be seen as having a greater responsibility to those with whom a professional relationship has been established than to other members of society.

Consequentialism

An alternative approach is that of consequentialism. Whereas in deontology there are a number of ethical principles, consequentialism has a single supreme principle, which requires that we should produce the best possible outcome. For the consequentialist, courses of action are not chosen on the basis of the various ethical principles which they either fulfil or contravene, but strictly in terms of the consequences which they are likely to bring about. Thus, the justification for insisting that the truth be told in a certain situation would be that to do so will produce better consequences for all concerned, rather than because this is dictated by an ethical principle such as respect for persons.

Indeed, there is a further contrast between deontology and consequentialism here. In the process of ethical decision-making, the consequentialist will choose the option which produces the best consequences, even if this involves breaching certain ethical principles which the alternative course(s) of action would have left intact. In the example given earlier, an occupational therapist using a consequentialist framework might deliberately exclude patients from the planning of their rehabilitation, or withhold certain information from them, if he or she thought that more patients would be successfully rehabilitated in this way. The fact that the patients' autonomy would be undermined would be outweighed by the overall good consequences brought about.

Within a deontological framework, things are the other way round. The deontologist will require that a certain course of action should be pursued because it observes one or more fundamental ethical principles, even if it produces less desirable consequences than the alternative. Thus, in contrast to a consequentialist approach, it would be argued that the truth should always be told to patients, even when demonstrably better consequences for all concerned would flow from the telling of a lie. McNaughton provides a vivid illustration of the difference between consequentialist and deontological approaches:

> Suppose a group of plane hijackers are threatening to kill all the passengers unless the British government agrees to hand over three of their opponents who have been granted political asylum in Britain. The government knows that, if the exiles are handed over to the hijackers, they will be tortured and executed. There is also good reason to believe that the hijackers will carry out their threat to kill the passengers since other members of their group have done so in past hijackings. (McNaughton, 1988:165)

The consequentialist solution, at least in terms of short-term considerations, would be to hand the exiles over to the hijackers. As there are probably several hundred passengers on the aircraft and only three exiles, this would represent a consider-able net saving of human life, and thus the best outcome in consequentialist terms. However, the deontologist would quite likely object to this, for several reasons. The asylum given to the exiles is effectively a promise to protect them, and to renege on this promise would constitute a serious breach of trust. Equally, sending these people to a certain death would be contrary to the requirements of non-maleficence. Moreover, it would be a clear example of using people purely as a means to an end, and thus contrary to the principle of respect for persons. In the final analysis, the deontologist would most likely claim that these considerations argue against handing the refugees over to the terrorists, even at the cost of an overall loss of life.

This does not mean, however, that deontologists are not concerned with producing good consequences – indeed, the principle of beneficence would seem to demand exactly this. Nor is it the case that consequentialists are wholly unconcerned with notions of justice, non-maleficence, etc. The essential point is that, for the deontologist, the acid test of a course of action is the intrinsic nature of the actions performed, and its conse-quences are ultimately of secondary importance. Likewise, the overriding consideration for the consequentialist is the outcome of a course of action, and the intrinsic nature of individual actions has no independent authority in the decision-making process.

In terms of consequentialist thinking, the individual should do whatever is necessary to secure the best possible outcome. This is likely to involve certain actions on the part of the individual him- or herself, but it may equally require steps to be taken to influence the actions of others; neither is intrinsically more important than the other. Here also, there is something of a contrast with deontology. The deontologist will regard agents as primarily concerned with what they themselves do; they are not responsible for the actions of others to the same degree.

Both consequentialism and deontology may generate rules of action. We have seen that, from a deontological perspective, respect for autonomy may give rise to the secondary principle of veracity. Observing this secondary principle is essentially equivalent to obeying a rule to the effect of 'always tell the truth'. Consequentialism may also generate a rule of action such as this, but the basis for doing so would be because of the beneficial effect of following such a rule, not because of its relationship to a more fundamental principle. Thus, consequentialist reasoning can dictate either that an individual action should be carried out on a specific occasion, or that this sort of action should be carried out on *all* relevantly similar occasions. These two approaches to consequentialism are known as act-consequentialism and rule-consequentialism respectively. In terms of justifying moral conduct, the crucial difference between the two is that act-consequentialism will endorse the course of action which will have optimum consequences in the case in question, whereas rule-consequentialism will support the action whose *consistent* performance would be for the best, even though its consequences on a particular occasion might be less than optimum. The function of rules will be considered further in Chapter 8.

A final note of caution is perhaps in order. The preceding discussion may suggest that deontological and consequentialist approaches will tend always to produce differing or conflicting conclusions in particular cases. This is by no means the case. Very often, consequentialists and deontologists will agree on the course of action which should be pursued; what will differ is the rationale and justification for their respective conclusions. In the case of Gary Bernstein described in the previous chapter, if the decision was taken to falsify the treatment record, this could be defended on consequentialist grounds; it might be argued that the benefit to Mrs Jaycynski from continued treatment would outweigh any undesirable consequences of falsifying the record. Equally a deontologist could argue for the same course of action, on the grounds that while there is a prima facie duty of veracity which would oppose falsification, the beneficence-based duty to continue treatment would in this case take priority. In fact, arguments could also be devised, on both consequentialist and deontological grounds, to oppose falsifying the treatment record. Thus, while consequentialism and deontology may differ considerably as forms of moral reasoning, they may or may not lead to different conclusions as to what moral action should be taken.

Virtue ethics

The two approaches to ethical decision-making which have been outlined above are both essentially concerned with what one *does*. The ultimate focus is on the actions which one performs. For some time now, certain philosophers have suggested that this is an incomplete account of morality, and that one should also be concerned with the sort of person one *is*, and the various character traits and motivations that one exhibits (Anscombe, 1958; Stocker, 1976). In other words, morality should be agent-centred as well as act-centred. We should value the virtue of discretion as well as actions which preserve confidentiality, benevolent dispositions as well as beneficent deeds, the virtue of honesty as well as actions of truth-telling, and so forth.

More recently, this question has received specific attention within health care ethics. The traditional approach based on the use of fundamental ethical principles and the use of analytical ethical reasoning has been criticized as being inadequate as an account of health care ethics. It has been objected that traditional approaches are too abstract and general, and do not adequately respond to the emotional and psychological dynamics of the health care context; as Nicholson comments: 'Real moral agents do not always work in the abstract; they exhibit emotions which get mixed up in decisions that are not always rational' (Nicholson, 1994:273). These traditional approaches have also been criticized for embodying a particularly 'masculine' approach to morality, and failing to reflect some of the concerns arising from feminist critiques (Sherwin, 1992), and the distinctively feminine nature of caring (Noddings, 1984). Thus, it is argued, the nature of professional work in health care requires a focus on the experiences of caring, compassion and suffering that characterize illness, and on the sorts of dispositions and virtues that are morally desirable in those involved in health care. This requires more than a simple analysis of which actions are right and which are wrong.

The approach that is suggested to remedy some of the alleged shortcomings of principle-based theories can loosely be described as one of virtue ethics. Its primary concern is with the sorts of character traits that one should display, one's motives, the feelings of duty and responsibility under which one should work, and the role of conscience and intuitive responses to particular situations.

This alternative model has its own problems, however. The first is that virtue ethics may simply be incomplete in the opposite way: 'Moral problems are frequently problems about what we should *do*. It is not obvious how, according to virtue theory, we should go about deciding what to do. What can this approach tell us about the assessment, not of character, but of action?' (Rachels 1993:176). Unless we can be sure that having the right virtues will ensure that one always performs the right action, which is surely not the case, there still seems to be a need for a specific focus on actions. There are many examples of situations in which people's intuitions or good intentions have led them to do things which we would regard as wrong. An additional problem is that the need for an explicit justification of moral conduct, as outlined in the following section of this chapter, seems much harder to fulfil within the virtue ethics approach. Appeals to character, conscience, or intuitions provide a less objective means of justification than a more analytical approach.

A further problem is that an uncritical focus on the cultivation of motives, virtues and character traits, to the exclusion of rigorous analysis of specific actions and their justification, may lead to a superficial and facile assumption that all that matters in health care is to be the 'right' sort of person. Brewin argues that the most caring doctor may be 'totally ignorant of academic ethics', and goes on to argue that the teaching of such ethics may

> discourage the firm 'captain of the ship' decisions that many frightened and confused patients (including many doctors when they are ill) and hospital staff will expect from the leader of a team in certain situations, however unfashionable and however unattractive to some ethicists.... Whatever the nature of the crisis, help comes from those who have the gift of good judgment, firm leadership, and common sense. (Brewin, 1993:161)

Such views are too imbued with specific social and professional values to serve as the touchstone of morally acceptable practice in health care within a pluralistic society. Although act-centred approaches are accused of being too abstract, they do help us to step outside some of our own values, perceptions and assumptions – which may not be shared by those for whom we care. This issue will be touched upon again in the discussion of advocacy in Chapter 9.

The answer to this dispute is perhaps not to replace one approach with the other, but to attempt to achieve a balance between the two, so that ethical decisions are not made without reference to the psychological, emotional and contextual features of the specific situation in which they occur. Indeed, this may be indispensable, if we agree that '[p]rinciples require judgment, which in turn depends upon character, moral discernment, and a person's sense of responsibility and accountability' (Beauchamp and Childress, 1994:462). In addition, while we may readily learn certain principles which tell us what we should or should not do, this may not be enough; it is the possession of certain moral attitudes, such as compassion and patience, that causes us to attach particular importance to such principles (Hunt, 1992; Dougherty and Purtilo, 1995). Purtilo strikes a useful balance when she distinguishes between two complementary elements of professional responsibility: 'responsibility as accountability', as assessed by the fulfilment of duties, and 'responsibility as responsiveness', which is

> measured by the agent's ability and willingness to respond – that is, his or her sensitivity to the needs of the occasion, flexibility, use of listening and communication skills, and creative approaches to the unique problem which is presenting itself at that moment. (Purtilo, 1986:580)

While we should give due concern to what we do, we should also seek to cultivate those qualities within ourselves that will facilitate and enhance the moral action that we take. The role of moral virtues in ethical decision-making is illustrated in Figure 2.2. The main features of deontology, consequentialism and virtue ethics are indicated in Table 2.2.

Justifying ethical decisions

There is a common view that ethics is just a matter of opinion, and that, consequently, there is no rational basis for deciding between competing views; one person's view is as valid as anybody else's. To be sure, many philosophers would admit that

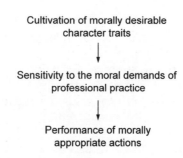

Figure 2.2 The role of moral virtues and character traits in ethical decision-making

there is indeed a subjective element in ethical reasoning, given that morality is a matter of values, which are subjectively held by individuals. It is hard to provide an objective account of why we hold the basic values that we do – they seem to be something that we feel, or perceive in an intuitive sense. Although there is often a high degree of moral consensus, we do not all hold precisely the same values, and this partly explains why there is rarely a *single* correct answer to an ethical conflict or dilemma.

However, to admit this is not to grant that ethical decision-making in its entirety is a purely subjective affair. The fact that values may be to a large extent individual does not reduce ethics to no more than a matter of opinion. What we are dealing with here are certain fundamental moral convictions, and these must be distinguished from matters of taste or personal bias:

> Taste involves matters of choice which are, though value-laden, essentially morally neutral. This, indeed, is what we *mean* by a matter of mere taste – that it pertains simply to preference, to matters without moral import. (Callahan, 1988:13)

Furthermore, we are obliged to provide reasons for our decisions on moral matters in a way that we are not when deciding on questions of personal taste. If we decide to drink tea rather than coffee, or to play water polo rather than croquet, there is no sense in which we are accountable for this choice. On the other hand, if we decide in a given situation to place the keeping of a promise to one person above the avoidance of harm to another person, it is quite reasonable to be asked to give our

Table 2.2 A simplified comparison of deontological, consequentialist and virtue ethics approaches to morality

Deontology	Consequentialism	Virtue ethics
Focuses predominantly on actions.	Focuses predominantly on actions.	Focuses predominantly on agents.
Concerned primarily with the observance of certain duties, based on basic moral principles of action.	Concerned primarily with the consequences of action.	Concerned primarily with the cultivation of moral dispositions or virtues.
Moral conflicts are settled by determining which is the 'weightier' duty.	Moral conflicts are settled by determining which alternative outcome is better for those concerned.	Moral conflicts are settled by determining which course of action exemplifies the more desirable moral character.
Particularly concerned with what the agent him- or herself does in a given situation; what the agent does is generally more important than what he or she prevents from happening.	Concerned with what anybody (the agent and others involved) does in a given situation, inasmuch as the agent can influence this; what the agent does and what he or she can prevent from happening are equally important.	Concerned with the moral virtues which the agent displays in his or her conduct; not primarily concerned with what the agent, or anyone else, *does*, per se (though it is recognized that good moral character will tend to generate morally good actions).
Attaches special moral weight to relationships between individuals, and the commitments which these imply.	Recognizes that relationships between individuals can be morally significant, but does not attach a special moral weight to these.	Attaches special moral weight to relationships between individuals.
Will countenance an outcome that is less than optimal if this is the only way to honour a fundamental moral duty.	Will countenance the breach of a fundamental moral duty if this is the only way to produce the optimal outcome.	Not primarily concerned with the honouring of moral duties or the production of good consequences.

reasons for doing so. Indeed, providing a justification for moral decisions is essential for a number of reasons:

1   It is important not only to make the correct decision at the end, but also to arrive at it by the right means. Otherwise, doing the right thing may be a matter more of luck than judgement, and sooner or later our luck will give out.
2   If we feel that an action is the right one for ourselves, we presumably feel that anybody else in the same situation should act similarly. It is only by explaining *why* we think our action was the right one that we are likely to convince others to act in the same way.
3   Very often in health care it is a matter of reaching a joint decision within a multidisciplinary team. This will frequently mean establishing a consensus among initially discordant views. Unless individual team members can give reasons for their own stance, it is unlikely that a consensus view will be reached.

Thus, morality inevitably involves a process of justification; but, we may ask, if there is a subjective element in ethics, how can we achieve any sort of objective process of justification? Here, it is important to realize that, although we cannot always justify our fundamental moral beliefs or principles according to any objective criteria, when we come to apply these principles to specific cases we are subject to three basic demands which are objective in nature.

The first of these demands is that the way in which we apply fundamental moral principles to a particular situation must be logical. When we seek to justify our decision in a certain case in terms of one or more of these principles, the steps we take in this justification must follow logically. Our particular judgements and actions are logically derived from certain rules, which are themselves derived from the principles which they seek to support, which in turn are further derived from certain wider ethical theories or systems of belief.

To take an example to illustrate this idea, you may wish to justify a case of truth-telling in terms of the principle of autonomy. Now, the basic ethical value that you attach to this principle cannot be conclusively invalidated or disproved. Indeed, others

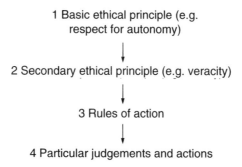

1 Basic ethical principle (e.g.
respect for autonomy)

↓

2 Secondary ethical principle (e.g. veracity)

↓

3 Rules of action

↓

4 Particular judgements and actions

Figure 2.3 A hierarchical process of ethical justification, based on the model proposed
by Beauchamp and Childress (1994:15)

may, from their own subjective viewpoint, disagree with the
moral weight which you attach to it, and relegate it in importance below certain other principles to which they attach
greater weight. Alternatively, they may question the sincerity
with which you hold this principle. However, it cannot be
dismissed out of hand on any objective grounds.

In contrast to this, the way in which you proceed to base a
particular course of action on the principle of respect for autonomy must stand up to objective scrutiny. Each of the hierarchical
steps in the process of justification illustrated in Figure 2.3 must
be defended. First, it must be argued that the secondary principle of veracity flows from the more basic principle of respect for
autonomy; a logical relationship must be shown between providing people with full and truthful information, and the protection
and promotion of their self-determination and freedom of action.
To move to the next step in the process, if you choose to formulate a specific rule of action concerning truth-telling in order to
uphold the principle of veracity (i.e. moving between levels 2
and 3 in Figure 2.3), you must demonstrate that this rule does
indeed bear a strong relationship to the principle it is designed
to fulfil; it is always open to somebody else to claim that a
somewhat different rule is more appropriate. Similarly, when
you implement this rule and take a specific course of action,
such as conveying certain items of information to a particular
patient or client (i.e. moving between levels 3 and 4), the onus is

once again on you to demonstrate that your action is in keeping with this rule. Your critics may claim that modifications to your course of action, e.g. in its timing or the manner you presented the information, would have allowed it to conform better to your rule, or they may argue that a different action would have been more in keeping with the rule.

Thus, although your adherence to the fundamental principle of autonomy cannot be refuted, the procedure whereby you derive a secondary principle from this principle, the way you extract a rule of action from this secondary principle, and how you justify a given action in terms of such a rule of action, are all areas where you can potentially be accused of being mistaken.

The second requirement is that this process of justification should be based on an accurate assessment of the facts. The decision-making process must be justified in terms of the empirical evidence, and it is always possible to misread this evidence. Perhaps what you took to be an apparent desire for information was in fact an implicit request to be shielded from unpleasant facts. As a result, your action may have done more to breach the patient's autonomy than to preserve it. Similarly, if you fail to obtain informed consent from a patient because you feel that he or she is not competent to give it, you must provide convincing evidence to show that the patient is indeed incompetent, in the same way as a course of treatment or rehabilitation must be based on a sound assessment of the individual's diagnosis or functional status.

The final requirement is that we should apply our ethical values and principles consistently. If there are two situations which are similar in all morally relevant respects, we are expected to reach much the same conclusion in each of them.

Indeed, it is worth noting how similar the demands of ethical decision-making are to those of such processes as clinical diagnosis, treatment planning, and goal setting. Throughout, there is a need for logical thought processes and close attention to the specific facts of the case in question, followed by the formulation of a systematic and coherent plan of action. It is possible, however, to take this analogy too far. Clawson (1994) draws a number of parallels between clinical and ethical decision-making. She endorses a system of ethical decision-making proposed by Barman and Hendrix (1983). It must be emphasized that Barman and Hendrix propose this model as a means of teaching ethical decision-making, and do not specifically advocate it as a procedure for reaching decisions in actual situations. Nonetheless, Clawson implies that it might be used in such a way. This system relies on the following principal steps: listing and ranking of values that are expressed in an ethical problem; listing alternative possible solutions to the problem, which are also ranked; and determining possible consequences of the preferred solution – again with ranking of these consequences. Finally, the participants are asked to indicate their degree of confidence in the stated solution on a four-point numerical scale (Barman and Hendrix, 1983:27–9).

To try to reduce ethical decision-making to so systematic a step-wise process is most likely a misguided enterprise. It is not clear that ethical values and principles can be weighed and ranked with the sort of quantitative accuracy implied in this model. It is important to accept that ethical decision-making is by its very nature a somewhat imprecise affair. While it is indeed important to weigh certain values against one another, this is not a mathematical process.

Conclusion

In this and the preceding chapter, a broad introduction has been given to the contextual and conceptual basis of ethical decision-making. Of necessity, this has involved examining a number of theoretical and at times seemingly abstract terms. However, an understanding of the basic concepts and principles of ethical theory is crucial for a critical understanding of concrete ethical conflicts. Otherwise, we risk an unreflective approach to ethical decision-making:

> [T]he doctor untrained in moral philosophy is prone to jump to ethical conclusions on the basis of gut feeling, without proper consideration of the issues involved. Illogical leaps are made, judgement is inappropriately swayed by emotive language, and inconsistent positions are adopted. (Toon, 1993:18)

It is now time to apply these ideas to specific applied ethical issues in therapy practice, and this will be the primary purpose of the remaining chapters of this book.

3

Truthfulness

In Chapter 1, we noted that many of the central issues of ethical concern to therapists are far removed from the high-profile topics that tend to receive greatest exposure in the media and other public arenas. Truthfulness is just such an issue. It rarely gives rise to dramatic, life-and-death consequences, but nonetheless has crucial ethical implications for therapy practice. In this chapter, the question of truth-telling will be discussed, and the allied topic of informed consent will be examined in the following chapter.

Telling the truth

It sometimes becomes apparent that the consensus of opinion on ethical matters has changed over time, and the question of truthfulness is an example of this. In early discussions of medical ethics, there tended to be very little reference to this topic. The notion of confidentiality was often mentioned – it is, for example, specified in the Hippocratic Oath – but truthfulness by and large was not. However, over the last twenty-five years or so, there has been more interest in telling the truth as part of the health professional's ethical obligations. Over this period, it seems that opinions have changed. For example, a study in the 1960s (Oken, 1961) looked at what physicians tell patients who have cancer, and found that 90 per cent of doctors routinely withheld the diagnosis from their patients. However, a study on the same issue in the 1970s found that doctors' attitudes had more or less reversed on this, and that they were in favour of telling the patient in the vast majority of cases (Novack *et al.*, 1979).

Nonetheless, the question of truthfulness is still one that attracts ethical controversy. It is one which therapists should take seriously, as, according to Bok, '[h]onesty from health professionals matters more to patients than almost everything else that they may experience when ill' (Bok, 1978:xvi). She also points out that health professionals may not realize the importance that patients attach to truthfulness:

> [M]any physicians talk about such deception in a cavalier, often conde-scending and joking way, whereas patients often have an acute sense of injury and loss of trust at learning that they have been duped. (Bok, 1978:xvi)

However, Barnitt (1994) found in a recent survey that truth-telling was identified as a source of ethical conflict by 34 per cent of occupational therapy respondents and by 30 per cent of physiotherapy respondents. This suggests that many therapists are well aware of the ethical implications of this issue.

Conceptual issues

Before we look in any detail at the specific ethical issues involved in telling the truth, we must briefly consider a few conceptual questions. The first of these is 'what is the truth?' Here, a distinction can be made between an 'objective' and a 'subjective' definition of truth. On the first of these, the truth is that which corresponds to the facts of the matter in a complete and accurate manner. It is a set of beliefs that bears a perfect relationship to reality. A subjective definition of truth, on the other hand, refers to the set of facts which the speaker *reasonably believes* to be an objective representation of reality.

In some areas of philosophy, such as epistemology (the theory of knowledge) or the philosophy of science, an objective definition of truth is of considerable relevance. In applied ethics, however, we are primarily concerned with what people believe to be the truth. A simple example will illustrate this. If I mention to you that I saw Peter at the airport yesterday – whereas, unknown to me, it was actually his twin brother Paul whom I observed – most people would hesitate to say that I was not telling the truth. My statement was factually inaccurate, but it was based on an honest belief. Of course, we prefer people to make factually accurate statements, but the main criterion as to a person's truthfulness is what that person sincerely believes to be the case.

This leads us to the next conceptual question: 'What is it to tell the truth?' There are two alternatives here:

1   To disclose all known details of the situation – 'the whole truth and nothing but the truth'.
2   To disclose a chosen proportion of the known details of the situation according to some standard or criterion. This might be justified on the basis that some details are sometimes more informative than all details.

Finally, there is the question: 'What is it *not* to tell the truth?' Here, there are four possibilities:

1   To say nothing, thereby withholding information which another person might be supposed to want and/or need.
2   To disclose some of the known facts but withhold others according to some standard or criterion (sometimes referred to as 'being economical with the truth'). This differs from the second means of telling the truth in terms of intent – there the motive was to inform, here it is to mislead.
3   To convey information known or believed to be contrary to the truth (the common meaning of 'lying').
4   To disclose some or all of the known details without any factual inaccuracy, but in such a way as to create misunderstanding: 'the truth can have the moral impact of a lie because it is meant to convey a false or misleading impression' (Veatch, 1981:223).

Hence there are different ways of telling the truth and different ways of failing to do so. A vexed question is whether or not the various ways of not telling the truth are morally equivalent. Acts of commission, such as lying, are often regarded as more reprehensible than acts of omission, such as withholding the truth. Thus, Beauchamp and Childress argue:

Deception that does not involve lying is generally less difficult to justify than lying, because it does not as deeply threaten the relationship of trust between deceiver and deceived. Underdisclosure and nondisclosure are typically still less difficult to justify. (Beauchamp and Childress, 1994:397)

Fromer provides a relevant example:

When a client asks 'will it hurt?' the therapist is obligated not to lie, but the expected intensity of pain need not be disclosed. Lying would destroy or damage the relationship of trust, whereas not fully disclosing the information would not. (Fromer, 1981:335)

Such a consequentialist distinction rests on the assumption that the deception is discovered. If, however, the deception is not revealed – or prior to the point at which it is – the consequentialist argument can be turned round: in cases of both lying and non-disclosure, the effect on the client's state of knowledge, and his or her subsequent actions, may be equivalent. Thus, if a therapist falsely states that a certain treatment is the only one available, as opposed to deliberately neglecting to draw the client's attention to other therapeutic options, the client is equally ignorant in both cases. Furthermore, the underlying motive of deception, and the contravention of the client's implicit expectation of honesty, are largely indistinguishable in each case. We should, therefore, be wary of assuming that withholding the truth is automatically less culpable than lying.

Why tell the truth?

There are a number of arguments put forward to support truthfulness in health care. Perhaps one of the strongest is based on the principle of respect for autonomy. Knowledge of one's situation, and of the choices that are open to one, is a precondition for autonomous action. To withhold information from patients is to deprive them of the basis of autonomous action. The patient who is not told his or her diagnosis, or is not informed of the various therapeutic options available, cannot make an informed choice of treatment. Other options are also foreclosed. For example, Downie and Telfer (1980:61) point out that 'a refusal to allow the patient to realize that he is dying cuts him off from the positive help nowadays available for such patients in the form of the hospice movement, or discussions with social workers specially trained for working in this sensitive area'. Similarly, in the case of inherited conditions such as Huntington's chorea, while there may be little in the way of therapeutic options, major decisions have to be made in respect of issues such as whether to have children; these cannot be made in ignorance of the diagnosis.

Alternatively, truthfulness can be grounded in the principle of respect for persons – to deceive people is to compromise their dignity and to treat them as less than a person in the full sense (Robinson, 1973; Benjamin and Curtis, 1986). This is particularly the case if the reason for the deception is the pursuit of a goal in which the person deceived has no stake.

A further consideration supporting veracity derives from the intrinsic nature of the therapeutic relationship. It can be argued that this is, by definition, a relationship of trust, and that truthfulness is therefore an essential component. In this connection, Veatch points to the contractual nature of the therapeutic relationship, and argues:

> It is the nature of lay–professional relationships that contractual bonds have been established requiring open communication. In such a situation, withholding information that it is reasonable to suspect the other person would find meaningful is a violation of that covenantal bond. (Veatch, 1981:225)

Similarly, Ellin (1982) argues that the professional–client relationship imposes a special duty of truthfulness on the practitioner. Interestingly, however, he restricts this to the case of lying. The purpose of this relationship, he argues, is to further the health-related interests of the client, and withholding information is a legitimate way of fulfilling such a purpose, and is compatible with the relationship of trust between professional and client. Lying, on the other hand, is a direct breach of this fiduciary relationship, and can therefore rarely be justified. Other arguments in favour of truth-telling take a more consequentialist form. Very often, the success of treatment or rehabilitation depends upon the full involvement and cooperation of patients, who must therefore understand the nature of their problems and the purpose of any therapeutic strategies implemented. Deception is inimical to this cooperative model of care. Furthermore, dishonesty is generally discovered sooner or later, and then destroys trust over a long period of time, outweighing the short-term benefit produced by the deceptive action. Once an instance of dishonesty has been revealed, all other information, which may be perfectly truthful, becomes suspect in the patient's mind (Rumbold, 1993). Even before it is discovered, such deception can create an intolerable   burden   on   the   patient–therapist   relationship. Communication becomes inhibited, for fear of divulging crucial items of information, and there is a general unease which makes it hard to deliver competent and effective care. This conspiracy of silence may spread to others, including the patient's relatives, with the result that the patient becomes profoundly isolated in his or her ignorance.

Finally, it can be argued that honesty and trustworthiness are key character traits which health professionals are expected to exhibit, and that to be other than truthful in one's dealings with patients is contrary to the caring ethos of health care, and exhibits a disposition which is incompatible with the role of the health care worker.

How can deception be justified?

A number of arguments are put forward to justify withholding the truth from patients. One of these is based on the fallibility of human knowledge and understanding. It claims that all knowledge is necessarily incomplete and uncertain, and that, even if the truth could be known in its entirety, patients would not be capable of assimilating such information. The conclusion reached is that there is no obligation to tell patients the truth, because the truth can never be known. This argument does not stand up to serious scrutiny, for two reasons. First, it confuses matters of morality with those of epistemology (Gillon, 1986). As we noted earlier, the issue at stake is what we believe to be the truth, not the truth in absolute terms. Indeed, the fact that the whole truth is not known is not really a reason for not telling the truth, for this very fact is part of the truth:

> [T]he issues to be judged are not concerned with the 'whole truth' but
> with the truthfulness of the nurse who, her colleagues might argue,
> should have told the patient truthfully that little was known about the
> treatment in question. (Schröck, 1980:142)

Second, the argument underestimates and mistakes patients'
ability to comprehend medical information. A number of studies
have suggested that doctors tend to underestimate the knowledge and understanding of laypersons (Pratt *et al.*, 1957;
McKinlay, 1975). Where lack of comprehension does occur, this
may be more to do with health professionals' use of jargon and
their failure to express information in terms appropriate to a lay
recipient (Faulder, 1985). Moreover, what is at stake is a capacity
to understand the *issues* involved and the *implications* of
certain medical details, not the technical details themselves. It is
not necessary to comprehend the detailed histopathology of
multiple sclerosis to appreciate the effect this condition will
have on one's life, the likely prognosis, the probable effectiveness of alternative treatments, etc.

Finally, this line of reasoning misconstrues the underlying
standard of adequacy that should govern the disclosure of information. What patients need is not necessarily full information,
but *enough* information, as judged by their particular decision-
making needs:

> There is a difference between being fully informed and adequately
> informed to make a decision, however. A patient is adequately informed
> if he or she has just enough relevant information to make a decision.
> (Kyler-Hutchison, 1988:286)

It follows from this, however, that if a patient cannot fully
understand, and therefore cannot make meaningful use of,
certain information, the need to disclose this information may be
correspondingly reduced. This may occur in cases of dementia;
by the time that the diagnosis can reliably be made, the patient
may no longer be able fully to comprehend it (Drickamer and
Lachs, 1992).

Another justification proposed for the withholding of information is that complete disclosure is somehow incompatible with
trust. In what seems to be an appeal to a form of virtue ethics,
Brewin (1985) argues that, instead of insisting that doctors

should practise high levels of disclosure, we should urge patients to repose high levels of trust in doctors. This argument begs important questions as to the relative values and priorities of patients and health professionals, and seems to ignore the fact that disclosure can itself be a means of building trust. It also underestimates the extent to which the patient can to some degree negotiate a standard of disclosure with the practitioner at the outset of their relationship.

Perhaps a more plausible argument in favour of deception is that this may be in the patient's best interests. Particularly in cases of life-threatening illness, it may be argued that knowing the truth causes unnecessary distress and destroys hope. In an article originally published in 1927, Collins expresses this argument from non-maleficence by giving the following advice:

> [T]he physician soon learns that the art of medicine consists largely in skillfully mixing falsehood and truth in order to provide the patient with an amalgam which will make the metal of life wear and keep men from being poor shrunken things, full of melancholy and indisposition, unpleasing to themselves and to those who love them. (Collins, 1988:139)

Indeed, it has been suggested that a poor prognosis may in some cases be a self-fulfilling prophecy (Cousins, 1980; Collins, 1988).

Against this, it can be said that the distress caused by receiving unpleasant news is often overrated, and it has been argued that patients' ability to cope with such news is frequently underrated (Wright, 1973; Goldie, 1982; Buckman, 1992; Higgs, 1994). Indeed, the anxiety, fear and emotional turmoil caused by ignorance or uncertainty can itself cause severe distress:

> Concealing medical knowledge from people makes them into captives in a bodily prison, trapped in a strange place full of menace, half real, half imagined. However pathological the body's state, such imagined terror is worse and more destructive than the knowledge which is carefully shared. (Campbell, 1984:29)

Crucially, when patients react badly to the receipt of bad news, this frequently has less to do with the factual content of the information than with the way in which it is communicated. Buckman (1992:8) suggests that 'unthinking and insensitive truth-telling is as deleterious, in its own way, as unthinking and insensitive truth-concealment'. It would seem, therefore, that the argument from non-maleficence does not operate against the breaking of bad news as such; it requires that the truth be told sensitively and compassionately. If it is done in this way, the distress caused by the receipt of unpleasant news can be minimized:

> Patients and families usually find ways to cope with and adjust to whatever picture reality paints, especially if clinicians deal with them sensibly, sensitively, and supportively. They rarely, if ever, recover from being deceived. (Scofield, 1993:344)

Bad news often removes hope, to be sure, but it also thereby removes uncertainty, and may provide a clearer basis for the individual's plans and decisions. It should also be remembered that just because patients may have given up hope for a cure or a full recovery, this does not mean that they cannot anticipate other aspects of their life – particularly those relating to personal and emotional fulfilment – with some sort of optimism. Thus, a woman who, following an injury to her knee, learns that the paralysis of her ankle dorsiflexors is irreversible must give up the hope of regaining full normal function of her leg. Equally, however, she can now take specific and positive steps to adapt her life accordingly; she can take up new leisure activities which will not be affected by her impairment, change her car or have it adapted, and make any necessary adaptations to her job as a teacher. Moreover, the whole argument from non-maleficence often rests upon a false premise – that distress equals harm. It may be that the anguish caused by unpleasant news may be an episode in a overall process of recovery which is ultimately beneficial to the patient (Anonymous, 1982).

The question of paternalism

Nonetheless, if we regard veracity as a prima facie, not an absolute, obligation, it may well be that there are cases in which other considerations, such as beneficence or non-maleficence, may override it (Thomasma, 1994). Such a view has a distinguished pedigree. The British philosopher Henry Sidgwick argued that 'where deception is designed to benefit the person deceived, Common Sense seems to concede that it may sometimes be right; for example, most persons would not hesitate to speak falsely to an invalid, if this seemed the only way of concealing facts that might produce a dangerous shock' (Sidgwick, 1907:316). Such a view is often referred to as *paternalism*. This is defined by Childress (1982:13) as 'a refusal to accept or to acquiesce in another person's wishes, choices, and actions for that person's own benefit', and by Dworkin (1972:65) as 'interference with a person's liberty of action justified by reasons referring exclusively to the welfare, good, happiness, needs, interests, or values of the person being coerced'.

Paternalism is based upon the notion that the health professional may in some instances be better able to judge patients' best interests than patients themselves. 'Strong' paternalism consists in the deliberate overriding of the competent wishes of another person, whereas 'weak' paternalism involves 'an action taken in the best interests of a patient who cannot give a fully informed consent for some reason, or who is not afforded the full possibility of free choice' (Pellegrino and Thomasma, 1988:7). A parallel distinction is one between 'hard' paternalism, where the patient's values are supplanted by those of the health professional, and 'soft' paternalism, in which values and goals are pursued which the patient is genuinely thought to share (Childress, 1982).

The essential feature of paternalistic action is that while the individual's interests are being furthered, his or her autonomy is overridden to a greater or lesser extent. Benjamin and Curtis use the term 'parentalism' to indicate the parallel with the parent–child relationship:

> Like the parent, the nurse will claim to be acting *on the behalf*, although *not on the behest*, of the patient; for, like the child, the patient is presumed unable to appreciate the connection between the nurse's behavior and his or her own welfare. (Benjamin and Curtis, 1986:53)

There are some cases which would seem to support a paternalistic approach to truth-telling. Thus, Singleton and McLaren (1995) describe the case of a young married couple involved in a major road traffic accident. The driver of the car dies from serious head injuries, and his wife undergoes major surgery, following which she is transferred to the intensive care unit in a critical condition. After 48 hours, she regains consciousness and asks the medical staff about her husband. However, fearful that the news of his death could reduce her chances of survival at this stage, they tell the woman that he is extremely ill until such time as she is able to cope with the information without adverse effects.

Why might we think that dishonesty was justified in a case like this? In the first place, it should be noted that the deception is temporary. The decision made is not one to deprive the patient of information permanently, but rather to delay its communication. In addition, given the circumstances in which the patient finds herself, it does not appear that being kept in ignorance significantly restricts her autonomy of action. Nor is it clear that the patient's own values and priorities, as far as these can be judged, are being deliberately disregarded; the paternalism occurring is 'soft' rather than 'hard'. The main consideration supporting deception, however, is probably the magnitude of the harm that might come to the patient. This suggests that the principle of non-maleficence could carry sufficient weight in a case such as this to override the prima facie duty of veracity.

In this instance, therefore, the use of a 'therapeutic lie' may be justifiable. However, in cases where the individual's autonomy is more seriously undermined by the telling of an untruth, or where there is evidence that an alien conception of the patient's 'good' is being imposed, or when deception is permanent rather than temporary, untruthfulness becomes harder to excuse, and the arguments favouring honesty will generally prevail. In any case, the burden of justification rests firmly upon the health professional (Bok, 1978), and individual cases in which concealment may be justified do not justify a general policy of deception (Campbell *et al.*, 1992).

As a note of caution, it should be remembered that arguments for concealment or deception that are advanced in the name of the patient's best interests sometimes turn out to conceal strategies for serving the interests of professionals themselves (Sim, 1986a).

How should relatives be involved?

It is fairly common practice in some units for a serious diagnosis to be disclosed to patients' relatives rather than to patients themselves. There may be two intentions underlying such a practice:

1 This may be in order to obtain information as to the patient's likely response to learning a piece of bad news; relatives can be assumed to know the patient's character and personality better than the health professional.
2 The motive may be to protect the patient from the distress that knowing the diagnosis is thought likely to cause.

The first strategy can strictly speaking be seen as overriding the patient's autonomy (in that the patient should be consulted as to whether his or her relatives are informed). However, if it is carried out in order best to determine how and when to disclose the diagnosis to the patient (rather than *whether* to disclose it), this may be felt to be justified. It could be argued that the initial, temporary overriding of the patient's right to information is a necessary step to respecting his or her autonomy in the long term. However, relatives' views on such an issue may be rather ambivalent, and apparently inconsistent. Maguire *et al.* (1996) found that whereas most relatives of patients with Alzheimer's disease felt that the patient should not be told the diagnosis, the majority also felt that they themselves would wish to know if they were to develop the disease. The second strategy, however, is likely to be performed *instead of* informing the patient. This is a much more serious breach of the patient's self-determination, and is correspondingly harder to justify against a charge of paternalism. Indeed, a recent study suggests that most cancer patients do not wish a relative to receive information without their consent, nor to determine what they themselves are told (Benson and Britten, 1996).

Requests for information and information waivers

On the basis of the arguments adduced in favour of veracity, it is reasonable to conclude that patients have a right to know the truth. However, this prompts two questions. The first of these concerns the extent to which the patient has to ask for the truth.

If the patient is seen as having a right to know, then somebody in the health care team has a duty to tell. The question arises, however: is this duty only invoked if the corresponding right to know is explicitly voiced? If the patient does not specifically request to know the truth, is it justified to keep silent? The problem here is that there may be things that the patient should know which he or she would have no reason to ask about. Rumbold argues that

> unless the patient clearly indicates that he does not wish to exert his right to information, then the professional has a clear duty to provide him with it. The onus does not lie on the patient to ask but on the professional to tell. (Rumbold, 1993:142)

Clearly, it is important to be attentive to any clues given by patients as to the amount of information they wish to receive. However, the underlying assumption should probably be that, in the absence of indications to the contrary, patients wish to know.

The second issue is more complex. The notion of a right to know the truth suggests that there is a corresponding right *not* to know – as was noted in Chapter 2, having a right to do something suggests that you also have a right not to do something. Does this mean that patients can insist on not being told the truth, i.e. that they can waive their right to the truth? This question faces a major logical difficulty. We may well accept that such a waiver is appropriate on the basis of the patient's autonomy. However, for the patient to refuse information is to deny the very basis of an autonomous decision. The individual cannot know the implications of the information which he or she is declining, and therefore cannot have a rational basis for such a refusal.

Ost recognizes this problem, and argues that the patient does not have the right to refuse information. To be autonomous requires one to be rational, but to refuse information in a case such as this cannot be rational:

> [T]he individual may be claiming to know what he cannot know prior to your disclosure of the information; namely, his evaluation of its relevance to his decision. But to claim to know what you cannot know is contradictory, i.e., irrational. (Ost, 1984:306)

Ost concludes that patients are duty-bound to receive information about their medical condition and alternative treatment options; to be autonomous is mandatory.

It should be said that a view such as this is opposed by some philosophers (e.g. Childress, 1982; Strasser, 1986), and it would seem to be in need of some qualification. Nonetheless, while supporting the notion of waivers in principle, Beauchamp and Childress suggest that a general practice of allowing waivers is dangerous, owing to the uncritical trust that some patients place in health professionals: 'the general acceptance of waivers of consent in research and therapeutic settings could make patients more vulnerable to those who would abbreviate or omit consent procedures for convenience, already a serious problem in health care' (Beauchamp and Childress, 1994:163). Three specific situations come to mind in which it might be unwise to accept a waiver:

1   Where there is a suspicion that the patient is under a misapprehension regarding some other fact, e.g. the refusal of information appears to stem from the patient's mistaken belief that he or she is terminally ill.
2   Where the individual is not likely to benefit, and may even be at risk, from a proposed procedure, e.g. certain forms of non-therapeutic research, or organ transplantation from a living donor (Childress, 1982).
3   Where the patient's decision to remain in ignorance may have implications for others, e.g. the patient's condition might pose a direct or indirect hazard to relatives, friends or colleagues at work. Curtin and Flaherty (1982) describe the case of a man with cancer of the liver who refused all information about this case, but continued to make major life plans which would have major implications for his family's welfare after his death.

However, where relatively minor items of information are concerned, and where the stakes for the patient are low, waivers should probably be respected. To do otherwise would seem unjustifiably paternalistic. Furthermore, even if it is established that a patient has a duty to obtain certain information, this does not in itself confer a right on the health professional to force this information upon the patient. To say that a patient has a duty to know something is a necessary, but not a sufficient, reason for imposing the information; this further step will generally need separate justification.

Finally, a practical problem should be noted. Appelbaum *et al.* (1987) argue that most patients will not be sufficiently knowledgeable to realize that they have a right of waiver over the receipt of information. Consequently, in order to promote patients' autonomy with respect to information waivers, the health professional may have to bring the possibility of such waivers specifically to their attention. However, patients may infer from this that they are *expected* not to want information, or that the professional is essentially reluctant to give it.

The role of the therapist

Most discussions of the ethics of truth-telling have focused on the role of the medical practitioner. There are, however, some specific problems facing the therapist in relation to this issue.

Therapists and nurses are generally in more frequent and prolonged contact with patients than doctors, and are therefore often asked for information regarding diagnosis, prognosis, and the like. The nature of much of the interaction that occurs between therapist and patient – functional assessment, explanation of treatment strategies, negotiation of treatment goals, etc. – is also likely to encourage questioning by the patient. Furthermore, Hailstone (1969) argues that, in a ward environment, the therapist may be perceived as somehow apart from the regular medical team, and is thus a likely recipient of the patient's anxieties and uncertainties.

Given this, the question as to who is authorized to provide patients with information is one which therapists find troublesome (Barnitt, 1994). Traditionally, the doctor is seen as the proper source of such information, but it is important to examine this assumption; is it based on anything other than a conventional view of professional hierarchies? There would seem to be two fundamental requirements for this process of communication:

1   The information should be accurate, and as complete as is appropriate in the circumstances.
2   The information should be conveyed clearly and effectively.

It is not clear that doctors necessarily fulfil these requirements better than other professional colleagues. With regard to certain details of the patient's condition, therapists may claim superior knowledge: the occupational therapist may be more able to assess the patient's ability to live independently on return to the community, and the speech and language therapist may be a better predictor of the likely resolution of a patient's aphasia. It would certainly seem to be the case that therapists are the best judges of the likely outcomes of their own interventions. Equally, if we turn to the manner in which information is transmitted, therapists can claim at least as much expertise as doctors in effective and sensitive communication with patients and clients.

Therefore, it is an open question who should properly disclose information to patients. The crucial requirement is that the person who does so should be competent. As was suggested above, there are many matters on which therapists are probably more knowledgeable than doctors. Conversely, there are topics on which the medical profession will usually have greater expertise – the nature of a surgical operation, the implications of a particular form of drug therapy, and so forth. Notwithstanding this, there are other pieces of information which, although they may originate from the doctor, pass into the common ownership of the health care team. Details such as the patient's definitive diagnosis, or the outcome of certain therapeutic procedures, are frequently well-established, uncontentious facts which are not in need of qualification or reappraisal. They may therefore be said to lie within the competence of various members of the health care team and, provided that sufficient information is known to provide further clarification and deal adequately with supplementary questions from the patient, the therapist may feel authorized to disclose these facts to a patient if the need arises.

When might this be necessary? Consider the following case:

> Dorothy Penfold is anxious to know the outcome of her oesophageal biopsy, and asks her physiotherapist, Fleur Jacobs, for the results. Fleur feels that Mrs Penfold has a right to know, and to this extent realizes that somebody has a duty to tell her. Ordinarily, however, this would be the

doctor, and Fleur therefore contacts the attending physician, Peter Medway, and asks him to give the patient the results of the test, which were positive. However, Dr Medway refuses to do so, arguing that it is unnecessary to burden Mrs Penfold with this information. Fleur argues that Mrs Penfold wishes to know the truth, and that she is psychologically capable of dealing with it. Moreover, knowledge of her prognosis would determine the plans that Mrs Penfold would make for her future. However, Dr Medway still refuses to disclose the findings.

Despite Dr Medway's apparent intransigence, there are further steps that Fleur can take. She can re-examine her own thinking on the matter. She can discuss the matter again with Dr Medway, and with other members of the team. She can encourage Mrs Penfold to press the matter herself with Dr Medway. Despite these efforts, the basic conflict may persist: the patient desires certain information, the therapist feels she should be given it, but the doctor refuses.

Often, in such situations, an individual health professional will accede to the doctor's 'authority', perhaps through notions of professional loyalty. In a study carried out by Schröck (1980), approximately 60 per cent of nurses asked to justify having lied to a patient or given an evasive answer, gave reasons in terms of 'doctor's orders' or 'ward policy'. Similarly, Sheehan (1985:333) argues: 'Whatever our personal views on the matter, there is also the question of the policy in operation in relation to the issue. If there is a "no tell" policy, then it is questionable how useful it would be for individual staff members not to respect the policy'. However, such an argument needs also to address the moral validity of the policy that has been arrived at. If the wrong decision has been made, the fact that it accorded with an accepted policy does not give it moral legitimacy.

In the final analysis, Fleur may feel that her obligation to respect the patient's autonomy outweighs feelings of loyalty to a fellow professional, and take it upon herself to inform Mrs Penfold of her diagnosis. Here, Fleur could be seen as acting in an advocacy role (see Chapter 9 for further discussion). This action may have unpleasant repercussions for herself professionally, which Fleur will have to face. However, it could be argued that this is more a prudential than a moral consideration, and does not detract from what she perceives to be her duty. Ultimately, she can argue that while she has responsibilities to her colleagues and to the institution for which she works, her primary responsibility is to her patients. A further argument which Fleur could advance to support her decision is that of personal integrity. Bok (1978:226) points out that '[t]he doctor's choice to lie increasingly involves co-workers in acting a part they find neither humane nor wise', and Fleur could argue that she has the right to refuse to be drawn into actions, dictated by another party, which she finds morally unacceptable.

Thus, the situation may arise in which the therapist feels morally impelled to disclose certain facts to a patient, even though it might initially seem that it is not his or her prerogative to do so. This might well involve contravening certain accepted protocols within the unit, or crossing what are regarded as normal professional boundaries. However, if it is felt that such steps are the only way to protect the patient's welfare, and provided that the therapist feels able to communicate the necessary information competently and effectively, such a course of action may be ethically justified.

Conclusion

The question of truthfulness is an important one for therapists, as it is likely to be encountered on a frequent and regular basis in everyday clinical practice. A number of arguments both in favour of and against telling the truth have been considered in this chapter. Those favouring honesty have generally emerged as stronger, and in any case there should be an initial presumption in favour of telling the truth; not to do so must be seen as an exception to this rule requiring special justification. This is not to say that therapists should go around telling clients the full details of their diagnosis, prognosis and general clinical situation in a reflex and indiscriminate manner. Before conveying important and potentially sensitive pieces of information, questions such as these should be asked:

- Is there reason to think that the client genuinely does not wish to have such information?
- Would it normally be my responsibility as a therapist to deliver such facts, and if not, am I nonetheless justified in doing so?

- Have I discussed the issue with other members of the multi-disciplinary team, and if so what light do their thoughts shed on the decision to tell?
- Do I have the appropriate communication and interpersonal skills, and the necessary background knowledge, to inform the client effectively?
- If the information is likely to have an unsettling or distressing impact, have preparations been made to assist the client in dealing with this?

4

Informed consent

Informed consent can be seen as a special case of the wider issue of veracity considered in the previous chapter. However, whereas truth-telling is essentially an ethical issue, informed consent gives rise to both legal and ethical issues. Under a number of legal systems, a failure to obtain valid consent can give rise to a civil action of negligence, or of trespass to the person (Brazier, 1992; Vines, 1996). Informed consent has implications for therapists in terms of both clinical practice and research, though only the former will be considered in detail in this chapter.

Many of the arguments supporting the importance of informed consent are the same as those already reviewed in favour of truthfulness. In addition to familiar notions such as the promotion of autonomy and the protection of the individual's status as a person, Capron (1974) describes four other functions of informed consent:

1 To avoid fraud and duress: 'to the extent that the physician–investigator engages the patient–subject in a comprehensive and comprehensible discussion of the proposed treatment, he reduces the likelihood of misleading or overbearing the patient–subject' (Capron, 1974:369).
2 To encourage self-scrutiny by health professionals; the consent requirement encourages health professionals to ensure the efficacy and scientific validity of their interventions.
3 To foster rational decision-making by patients as well as professionals.
4 To involve the larger society in the debate, and thereby make the public more knowledgeable, about clinical practice and research.

Elements of informed consent

Informed consent may be defined as: 'the voluntary and revocable agreement of a competent individual to participate in a therapeutic or research procedure, based on an adequate understanding of its nature, purpose, and implications' (Sim, 1986b:584). Figure 4.1 shows how informed consent can be analysed into its constituent elements. Each of these must be present to a satisfactory degree if consent is to be valid.

Disclosure

This refers to the account provided by the health professional. Traditionally, it has been argued that the adequacy of this account should be judged by a *medical standard*, such that health professionals themselves should decide what patients need to know in order to be adequately informed (Ingelfinger, 1972, 1980; Garnham, 1975; Tobias and Souhami, 1993). In the UK and most states of the USA, this is the standard used by the law. More recently, two alternative standards have been proposed. The first of these is the *prudent patient* standard, which determines the adequacy of disclosure in terms of what a reasonable person would wish to know. In Canada and some states of the USA, the prudent patient standard has achieved legal recognition (Brazier, 1992; Mason and McCall Smith, 1994). An objection to the prudent patient standard is that 'information which is material to a decision may depend to some extent upon the idiosyncrasies of the particular patient' (Strong, 1979:196). Hence, the other alternative standard is known as the *subjective*

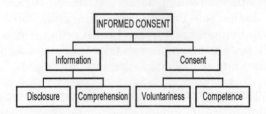

Figure 4.1 The constituent elements of informed consent

standard, and is related to the information needs of the individual patient, rather than those of the generic patient which form the basis of the prudent patient standard. This is in keeping with the observation in the previous chapter that the standard of adequacy for information should be relative to the needs of the individual.

An important consideration regarding disclosure is that information should be provided not only on the intervention that is being proposed to the patient, with its various risks and possible benefits, but also on alternative interventions which, while they may not be the treatment of choice from the professional's perspective, may nonetheless be more acceptable to the patient. Of relevance here is the choice between active treatment and self-management. Many patients might prefer to engage in exercises or other activities which can be carried out at home rather than attend for treatment at an out-patient facility (i.e. ambulatory care) – even though the latter might be somewhat more effective, or produce an improvement in a shorter period of time. However, it is only if both alternatives are presented that the patient can make such a choice.

Comprehension

Whereas disclosure has to do with the details imparted by the professional, comprehension concerns the message received by the patient; disclosure relates to the *sufficiency* of information, comprehension to its *intelligibility*. Another way of looking at this is that disclosure concerns the *content* of the information, whereas comprehension has to do with the *form* in which it is delivered. Clearly, these are joint requirements; a high standard of disclosure must be accompanied by adequate understanding by the recipient. As Lesser points out, the standard of comprehension must be patient-based: 'the right to be informed must be a right to be informed in a way that one can understand; it is for the professional to adapt to the layperson as far as possible' (Lesser, 1991:156). Equally, Purtilo (1993) stresses that the key issue is not so much the nature or extent of the information that is disclosed, but the *use* that the patient is able to make of such information.

For comprehension to occur, the patient must clearly understand the nature of the events or procedures to which consent is
being sought. However, it is less often appreciated that the
patient should further realize that a specific process of giving
agreement is occurring; it is a question of being aware *that* one
is authorizing as well as understanding *what* one is authorizing
(Faden and Beauchamp, 1986).

Voluntariness

Consent should be given without undue pressure, influence,
inducement or coercion. It has been suggested that there will
always be some pressure on the patient to consent (Ingelfinger,
1972; Fromer, 1981), perhaps reflecting the status differential
that exists between professional and patient, or arising from the
patient's desire to please or show gratitude. Of greater concern
are those instances in which pressure is deliberately applied to
the client – albeit implicitly or covertly – to agree to a certain
form of treatment. In psychiatric settings, an informal (i.e. voluntary) patient might be persuaded to comply with therapy under
the implied threat of a compulsory treatment order.

Consent that is not freely given is both legally and ethically
suspect. However, as will be discussed shortly, the boundary
between persuasion and manipulation or coercion is sometimes
indistinct.

Competence

This essentially refers to the patient's ability to reach a rational,
autonomous decision. Where there is impairment of competence, this may be permanent (e.g. learning disabilities,
irreversible coma), temporary (e.g. young children, persons
under the influence of alcohol or drugs, or those in an acute
confusional state), or intermittent (e.g. periodic amnesia, or a
mental illness characterized by alternating periods of confusion
and lucidity). Competence must be distinguished from the
ability to comprehend; an individual with a receptive disorder
may have difficulty in understanding the information being

conveyed, but may be fully capable of forming rational decisions on the basis of such information as he or she is able to assimilate. It should also be stressed that competence is contextual rather than global, and relative to a particular decision (Buchanan and Brock, 1989). The fact that a person may be incompetent in one area of life should not be extrapolated to others: 'a person who is incompetent to decide about financial affairs may be competent to decide to participate in medical research' (Beauchamp and Childress, 1994:134).

Furthermore, the degree of competence required may vary with the implications of the decision concerned; a lesser degree of competence may be acceptable in relation to decisions whose consequences for the patient are likely to be relatively trivial, whereas far more stringent criteria may apply when matters of more significance are at stake (Buchanan and Brock, 1989; Drane, 1991). Thus, a patient with some degree of cognitive and emotional disturbance following a head injury may be deemed competent to agree to a session of dressing practice or to the provision of feeding aids, but not sufficiently competent to consent to being rehoused, or to some other intervention which is likely to have irreversible effects.

Assessing competence

Attempts have been made to establish objective tests of competence (Roth *et al.*, 1977; Appelbaum and Roth, 1982; Appelbaum and Grisso, 1988; Wear, 1993). These are beset by problems. One of the difficulties is that such tests tend to seek a discrete threshold judgement as to whether a patient is competent, whereas competence probably lies on a spectrum; establishing the point at which to draw the line is problematic. Furthermore, as has just been noted, it may well be that the line should be drawn at different points in respect of different sorts of decisions to be made within a person's life.

Most cases in which therapists are required to obtain consent probably do not call for formal tests of competence. Nonetheless, there are a number of situations in which determining the competence of a patient or client may be less than straightforward.

First, therapists who are treating patients with certain cognitive or behavioural problems have to decide if these deficits prevent the individual from making a rational choice as to whether or not to accept treatment. Many of these patients are elderly; Murphy (1988) estimates that two thirds of the elderly people treated by psychiatrists are unable to give real consent to treatment.

Few such cases are clear-cut. Bailey and Schwartzberg (1995) describe the case of Mrs Ciarrelli, who is suffering from early-stage Alzheimer's disease, and is beginning to experience confusion and engage in unsafe behaviour when left at home during the day while her son and daughter-in-law are at work. Her family feel that Mrs Ciarrelli would benefit from occupational therapy, but she refuses to let the therapist visit her. In a case such as this, at what point in the progress of the disease does the client's disorientation render her incompetent to make autonomous decisions? Any such judgement should be made in the light of the unfortunate tendency to assume that incompetency is an inevitable accompaniment of old age (Muir Gray, 1994). Furthermore, if it is felt that Mrs Ciarrelli is indeed incompetent to a certain degree, to which areas of her decision-making does this apply?

At the extreme, some patients who are a danger either to themselves or to others can be administered treatment against their will, under such legislation as the UK Mental Health Act 1983 (Mason and McCall Smith, 1994) and various legal provisions in the USA (Miller, 1991). However, it is specifically emphasized in the document *Consent for Occupational Therapy* (COT, 1993:3) that incapacity to consent 'is not automatically to be implied by reason of the consumer's mental disorder, or because the consumer is subject to a section of the Mental Health Act'. In other cases, people with mental health problems may be attending as informal patients, and to that extent are receiving treatment voluntarily, but are nonetheless subject to interventions which may seem to be against their wishes. Eating disorders such as anorexia nervosa are managed in a variety of ways, but in some cases the individual's eating behaviour is conditioned by a form of behavioural therapy (Knibbs, 1993). The following example illustrates the ethical problem that can arise:

Carolee Clifton is a 17-year-old woman suffering from anorexia nervosa who, at the instigation of her parents and with her own agreement, has been admitted to the psychiatric in-patient unit. Here she undergoes a programme of behaviour modification, consisting of a system of reinforcements and sanctions designed to re-establish normal eating habits. On many occasions, Carolee protests when sanctions are carried out, and often weeps or shouts at members of staff. However, her protests and refusal to cooperate are largely ignored.

In a case such as this, there may be a fundamental ambiguity as to the nature and extent of the patient's consent. Although she has consented to the treatment programme as a whole, she appears not to be consenting to various components of the treatment process. Given that Carolee is not subject to a compulsory treatment order, it can be assumed that she is competent to consent, and no doubt her wish to discharge herself from the programme would be honoured, perhaps after some persuasion not to do so. However, there might also be a feeling that resistance to specific aspects of therapy should not be taken at face value. The staff may argue that these are simply manifestations of the process of denial that often characterizes anorexia nervosa, and might further claim that Carolee's initial consent to treatment in some way authorizes the overriding of her subsequent apparent objections or refusals, by means of a form of 'precommitment' (Dresser, 1984). A fine judgement may be required between imposing a form of behavioural control that is legitimately part of the treatment 'contract' to which the patient is party, and the need ultimately to respect her autonomous right to refuse consent and withdraw her participation.

A second situation in which competence may be felt to be doubtful is in the early stages of severe physical disability. The psychological impact of the onset of disability may be felt to have temporarily compromised the individual's competence to a certain extent. A patient who has experienced a spinal injury and is beginning the process of active rehabilitation may be reluctant, or even refuse, to participate in the programme of activities which the therapists have drawn up. Equally, a person who has undergone a non-elective amputation following a serious accident may decline to cooperate in the post-operative treatment regime. As Scofield (1993:342) suggests, this sort of case may raise the question: 'Is it the trauma or the patient talking?' Caplan maintains that this sort of situation may justify some degree of paternalism. He argues that

> rehabilitation professionals may be justified in overriding or ignoring the autonomous wishes of patients upon entry to a specialized unit for treatment if there are reasons to believe that the person either has not adapted to the traumatic realities of impairment, or that the patient will require some time to fully appreciate the possibilities available for coping with and adapting to chronic impairment. (Caplan, 1988:315)

Caplan bases this view on the argument that paternalistic intervention in the short term may be the best way of promoting the client's long-term autonomy. However, the problem remains as to how we, as 'outsiders', are to decide that the client's short-term wishes are in some sense at variance with his or her long-term goals. Even if they are, it is not self-evident that long-term considerations automatically take precedence. The client's social, educational and cultural background may be such as to give a different weight to short-term goals from that which most health professionals would think appropriate. Furthermore, it should be remembered that professional definitions of notions such as 'coping' or 'adjustment' tend to embody assumptions and preconceptions which are not shared by disabled people themselves (French, 1994).

Nonetheless, despite such reservations, Caplan's view is basically plausible, and there may indeed be cases in which some degree of 'substituted judgement' on the part of the therapist is justified. However, given the uncertainty that must exist as to what are the client's 'true' wishes, it is important not to take any paternalistic actions which will foreclose future options which the client might wish to take. Just as the individual's inability to make fully rational decisions is only temporary, so any actions taken on his or her behalf should not be irreversible in their effect.

Another situation in which competence may be uncertain is when an individual is presently in pain or distress. Physiotherapists face such situations when encouraging patients to perform exercises which may cause them discomfort, or when it is felt necessary to carry out endotracheal suction on a seriously ill but conscious patient. Pain and distress are fairly normal features of everyday life, and the assumption that individuals cannot respond rationally in such circumstances should be resisted. Nonetheless, as in the previous case, it is reasonable to think that the immediacy of patients' discomfort may distort their priorities; many therapists have subsequently been thanked by patients for having 'pushed' them when they were unwilling to cooperate. Here, the therapist must ensure that adequate attention is given to the various ethical values at stake. Were the therapist to discontinue treatment at the first 'No, thank you' from the patient, this would be to abrogate the duty of beneficence. Some degree of persuasion would clearly seem to be called for. However, with each refusal, the patient is giving an increasingly firm indication of his or wishes. Unless there is reason to think that such refusals are not autonomous, it is likely that a stage will be reached where the therapist feels that further persuasion will spill over into coercion, at which point the patient's autonomy will be overridden. At this point, unless a strong paternalistic stance is to be adopted, the patient's choice should be honoured. Moreover, even once the patient's desires have been acceded to, there is a responsibility continuously to monitor the patient's wishes, to ensure that the desire not to be treated is an enduring one.

The final category of patient in whom the assessment of competence may be less than clear is children. Although an age is set at which children are regarded as legally competent to consent to medical treatment (in the UK this is currently 16), this does not necessarily answer the moral question as to when children's choices should be regarded as autonomous. Indeed, since the Gillick case, the UK legal system has recognized that, viewed individually, children below the age of 16 may well be competent to make important medical choices for themselves. In addition, work by Alderson (1990, 1993) has indicated that the ability of children to make reasoned and autonomous choices tends to be markedly underestimated. She comments: 'Narrow meanings of knowledge and maturity are used to justify withholding information from children and then to label them as ignorant and exclude them from sharing in decisions' (Alderson, 1993:193).

When judging the competence of a patient to consent to treatment, therapists should take a conservative approach, i.e. they should only classify clients as incompetent on the basis of strong and unambiguous evidence. Thus, they should work on the assumption that all clients should be assumed to be competent until and unless they are shown to be incompetent, not vice versa. A divergence of the patient's values and priorities from those of the therapist, or the mere fact of non-compliance, should certainly not be taken as evidence of irrationality or incompetence. That having been said, Venesy (1994) points out that if the patient's decisions or desires alter substantially and repeatedly over a short period of time, this may suggest some degree of incompetence. She further alerts us to decisions which seem to be at variance with the patient's known values and goals – these too may warrant further examination.

Where incompetence is deemed to be present, this should only influence therapy to the extent that is strictly appropriate – the client should not thereby be excluded from any part in his or her care:

> Even in cases where mental functioning is clearly impaired, a morally sound approach dictates enlisting the participation of elderly patients as much as possible in decisions regarding their own care and treatment. (Macklin, 1982:128)

Obtaining consent

There are a number of forms that consent may take. *Express* consent is where the individual explicitly indicates his or her agreement, either orally or in writing. *Implied* consent occurs when the individual does not specifically indicate agreement, but performs some action which suggests that consent is forthcoming. Brazier (1992) gives the example of a patient visiting an accident and emergency department with a bleeding wound; the act of attending the department constitutes implied consent to the cleaning and bandaging of the wound. A more equivocal form of consent is *tacit* consent, which is inferred from the individual's failure to dissent. Finally, in the case of patients who are permanently or temporarily incompetent, consent may be *presumed*. Alternatively, in such cases *proxy* consent may be obtained from a relative or guardian (Banja, 1986). According to Barnitt and Fulton (1994), the form that consent should take is a matter that gives rise to concern among therapists. The legal situation is likely to vary somewhat from country to country, and there will often be specific institutional requirements. Nonetheless, implied consent is probably sufficient in most cases, because there are very few interventions carried out by therapists which do not require active cooperation from the patient; the act of participating in the activities concerned can usually be taken as consent. This, of course, is not to say that a detailed explanation on the part of the therapist is unnecessary; it merely suggests that explicit agreement on the part of the patient may not be required. In speech and language therapy in particular, receptive and/or expressive difficulties may mean that implied or tacit consent is the best that can be obtained from the client. Of course, this does not remove the need to provide an explanation and ascertain the client's agreement as far as this is practicable.

In other instances, express consent may be advisable. Such cases would include those in which there is a chance of discomfort, or some risk of hazard (particularly if these are not readily apparent). Techniques that are invasive also fall into this category (Barkes, 1979), and Barnitt and Fulton (1994) point out that such procedures need not merely be physical ones, such as acupuncture; certain verbal treatment strategies may be perceived by clients as psychologically invasive. Equally, activities or intimate procedures that may cause the patient or client embarrassment or loss of dignity may call for express consent. In physiotherapy, certain manipulative procedures are carried out without the active participation of the patient, and are such that the patient is not capable of preventing them from occurring. In such cases, it is hard to demonstrate implied or tacit consent, and express consent is probably advisable on both legal and ethical grounds (Delany, 1996; Sim, 1996a).

The question that arises next is whether this express consent should be oral or written. It should be said that, in the UK at least, there is no difference in the legal status of the two forms of consent. However, it is easier to demonstrate that written consent has been obtained; hence, Purtilo (1984) suggests that written consent may at times be advisable. Against this, it could be argued that asking the individual to give consent in writing might place the patient–therapist relationship on a rather legalistic footing, something which many therapists would regard as undesirable. The College of Occupational Therapists gives the following advice:

> Oral consent is acceptable in the majority of occupational therapy inter-
> ventions and the way in which oral consent is expressed shall be
> recorded in the consumer's notes....Written consent must be requested
> if substantial risk is involved in the recommended occupational therapy
> intervention. (COT, 1993:2)

Although written consent may have certain advantages in terms of legal evidence, therapists should be wary of assuming that it is superior to oral consent in other ways. In particular, the standard of the communication process involved in gaining consent is not necessarily related to its being written as opposed to oral:

> Consent forms simply document that some discussion has taken place.
> The quality and clarity of the information which is given is what is
> paramount: that is more important than simply having a signature on a
> piece of paper. Consent forms are evidence of a process not the process
> itself. (BMA, 1993:9)

Nor is the presence of a signed consent form evidence that the moral demands of consent have been met:

> That there is a completed consent form implies only that the physician
> has made some effort to communicate with the patient, but its existence
> does not guarantee fulfillment of ethical and legal responsibilities.
> (Sulmasy *et al.*, 1994:193)

One of the themes pervading recent discussions of informed consent is whether it is properly viewed as an event or a process. In other words, is it a discrete episode that occurs at a given time in the relationship between therapist and patient, or is it part of an ongoing dialogue between the two parties, throughout the patient's treatment? Recent thinking has tended to swing from the former view to the latter. Wear (1993) is probably right, however, to underline the virtue of having both an event and a process element in informed consent. In favour of the event element, he points out that 'such a one-shot intervention has the advantage of signaling to the patient that a significant choice is at hand, rather than allow such choices to be obscured or overlooked within some more free flowing process' (Wear, 1993:80).

This reinforces Faden and Beauchamp's (1986) idea, referred to above, that the patient should know *that* he or she is giving authorization. On the other hand, viewing consent as a process ensures that the therapist is constantly attuned to possible misunderstanding or changes of mind on the part of the patient. The patient's cognitive, behavioural and emotional responses to illness or disability develop and alter over time, and cannot be adequately captured at a single moment. More fundamentally, viewing consent as a process recognizes the fact that a continuous negotiation of goals usually characterizes the relationship between patient and therapist, in contrast to the short-lived interaction that often occurs between patient and medical practitioner in more acute settings. The specific nature of therapy suggests, therefore, that a process element within informed consent is crucial.

Consent and compliance

The notion of consent is closely linked to that of compliance. To consent to a course of action involving or affecting oneself is to submit to a plan that has been largely predetermined by another. Accordingly, the traditional model of consent assumes that the health professional is the initiator of therapeutic options, and the patient occupies a passive, subordinate role in this process. Such a perspective has been reinforced by the idea of the 'sick role' advanced by sociologists such as Parsons (1951, 1972). This formulation of the rights and obligations of the sick person imposes a responsibility on the patient to cooperate with technically competent care, in return for a temporary release from usual social duties. In contrast to this, modern client-centred models of therapy regard the client as an equal partner in the setting of therapeutic goals, and reject the view of the professional as active initiator and the patient or client as passive recipient of care. This modern model of care is especially appropriate to cases of chronic illness, for which the traditional sick role, with its focus on acute illness, does not adequately cater (Gallaher, 1976).

The concept of compliance is a problematic one, containing fundamental and value-laden assumptions as to the appropriate relationship between patient and practitioner (Holm, 1993). It is not surprising, therefore, that patients' own conceptualization of 'compliance' is likely to differ considerably from that of health professionals (Stimson, 1974; Roberson, 1992).

A further issue connected with the notion of compliance is the assumption that non-compliance is necessarily a problem. Indeed, Coy (1989a) suggests that even when non-compliance achieves a better medical outcome than would have come about through compliance, health professionals still tend to view such non-compliance as problematic! Additionally, the problem of non-compliance is seen as residing firmly within the patient, rather than being a product of the relationship that exists between patient and practitioner. Discussions of non-compliant behaviour tend to focus on means of overcoming or reversing such resistance, rather than on the prior question as to whether the patient ought to comply with treatment in the first place. The root of such thinking is perhaps the orientation of benefi-cence with which health professionals tend to work. The treat-ment plans that practitioners draw up are geared to providing the best possible outcome for the patient or client, as judged by the professional. Any behaviour that frustrates the realization of these plans is seen as impeding the patient's best interests, and is therefore deemed to be undesirable and problematic. According to Swain (1995), therapists may find it hard to accept that patients should be allowed to make choices that are seen as harmful to them. However, we should remember that to say that a situation is psychologically or emotionally troublesome is not necessarily to say that it is *morally* problematic.

If the focus is shifted to autonomy, however, a different picture emerges. Now the moral priority moves from the patient's inter-ests as defined by the professional to the patient's own autonomously formulated interests. If these self-defined interests conflict with those of the professional, non-compliance becomes a perfectly rational response, and it is the practitioner's paternalis-tic action that becomes problematic. Therapists and other health professionals often find it hard to give priority to the patient's wishes and intentions in this way because this seems to deny their own professional expertise. They feel that their own specialized education and training gives them a special qualification to determine what should be done to further a patient's health, just as a lawyer or an accountant has a distinctive expertise in relation to an individual's legal or financial affairs. This, however, is to misunderstand the nature of professional expertise. In particular, professionals tend to generalize this expertise beyond its legitimate confines (Veatch, 1973). Freidson provides a useful analogy:

> [W]e can all agree that how a road is to be built is a technical question best handled by engineers and other experts. But whether a road *should* be built at all, and *where* it should be located are not wholly esoteric technical questions. There are certainly technical considerations which must be taken into account in *evaluating* whether and where a road should be built, but engineering science contains no special expertise to allow it to decide whether a road is 'necessary' and what route 'must' be taken. (Freidson, 1970:336)

In other words, while health professionals can give an expert opinion on how best to *attain* a certain therapeutic goal, and on whether such a goal is realistic in practical terms, they have no specific authority in determining what this goal should *be* in the first instance. Hence, any view that compliance is necessarily a good thing presupposes a certain beneficence-based view of the patient's good.

Nor, however, is compliance necessarily a *bad* thing. As Coy argues:

> Compliance, in and of itself, is value neutral – it is neither good nor bad. If a patient complies with medical advice, it does not follow that the patient's autonomy has been diminished, that the patient obeyed unquestioningly, or that the patient was manipulated. What makes a particular instance of compliant behavior good or bad, from the moral point of view, are the circumstances that lead to the compliance. If a patient is coerced or manipulated into compliance – and hence, is not allowed free choice – then, from the moral point of view, the compliance is objectionable. On the other hand, patients can, and do, autonomously choose to comply with medical advice. (Coy, 1989b:53)

This quotation underlines the fact that while compliance may result from paternalistic activities of persuasion on the part of health care providers, it may also be a perfectly autonomous choice. A competent individual can make a conscious and rational decision to delegate the major portion of decision-making concerning his or her medical care to a professional, and may gain a sense of reassurance and confidence through having done so (Ingelfinger, 1980). It is therefore not automatically the case that the notion of compliance 'diminishes any notion that human beings are free to determine their actions' (Guccione, 1988a:70); it all depends upon the source of compliance.

It would seem, therefore, that from the point of view of autonomy, it is not enough simply that the act of consenting should be voluntary and uncoerced; it is necessary also to go one stage further back and look closely at the course of action to which consent is being sought. Is it the outcome of a genuine negotiation between practitioner and client, or is it 'a mere formality in which [health care providers] list acceptable goals (from the professional point of view), then ask patients to prioritize them' (Coy, 1989b:58)? Above all, therapists should resist the temptation of regarding the consent process as a means of reinforcing compliance; this is to put the cart before the horse. Rather, consent should be seen as a means of honouring the patient's self-determination, and compliance, or indeed non-compliance, will follow as appropriate.

If the desire for compliance on the one hand, and the need to respect the individual's autonomy on the other hand, are kept in a proper balance, professional interventions can be ethically sound and at the same time clinically effective:

> Patients rarely become invested in agendas that they have neither participated in setting nor had explained to them. On the other hand, patients and families who have a central role in determining treatment goals are far less likely to undermine therapy and more likely to perceive learned skills as relevant enough to carry with them upon discharge. (Scofield, 1993:343)

Conclusion

Informed consent is a key ethical issue within therapy. While the *formal* acquisition of consent may be necessary only on fairly rare occasions, there is a constant need to ensure that apparently insignificant therapeutic activities are carried out with the full agreement of those whom they most affect.

The issue of consent provides a vivid illustration of the tension that may exist between the principles of autonomy and benefi- cence, and the need to ensure that some sort of balance is kept between these two values. Equally, it helps to clarify what should be understood by the term 'compliance', and to appraise some of the assumptions which underlie it. The concern that currently exists for joint goal-setting and the use of patient-defined outcomes (Ahorny and Strasser, 1993; Rigge, 1994) will perhaps help to guard against the sort of paternalism that may obscure the need for a model of consent based on autonomy.

5

Confidentiality

In Chapter 3, it was noted that the relationship between the
therapist and the client is one built on trust, and that fidelity is a
character trait associated with those in the caring professions.
Hence, there is a moral presumption in favour of truthfulness on
the part of the therapist. However, these features of the therapist–client relationship that support the disclosure of information to the patient also support its withholding from other
parties. Thus, Thompson (1979:60) argues that confidentiality is
'an essential moral pre-requisite of the contractual relationship
into which patient and doctor enter' and Koehn (1994) argues
that for professionals to enjoy any form of moral authority they
must be seen to be trustworthy. To a large degree, therefore,
truthfulness and confidentiality are two sides of the same coin.

In addition to its links with the character trait of fidelity, confidentiality is intimately associated with that of discretion, which
is similarly regarded as central to the role of the health professional. Exhibiting such dispositions is part of what it means to
fulfil the vocation of a therapist.

Recent discussions of the ethics of occupational therapy have
emphasized the centrality of confidentiality to the client–practitioner relationship (Thompson, 1990; Barnitt, 1993; Bailey and
Schwartzberg, 1995; Sim, 1996b). Equally, codes of ethics within
the therapy professions consistently draw attention to the importance of respecting privileged information, for example:

> Speech therapists must maintain professional confidentiality with regard
> to their patients, and must refrain from disclosing information about a
> patient which has been learned directly or indirectly in a professional
> capacity. (CST, 1988:3)

Beyond any essential sharing of information with professional colleagues, occupational therapists must safeguard confidential information relating to consumers. (BAOT, 1990:3)

Information relating to the physical therapist–patient relationship is confidential and may not be communicated to a third party not involved in that patient's care without the prior written consent of the patient, subject to applicable law. (APTA, 1991)

Confidentiality and privacy

Confidentiality has close affinities with the concept of privacy. However, the two are by no means synonymous. Privacy has to do with access to one's fellow citizens, both physically and in terms of information concerning them. These two forms of privacy are distinct; few of us have direct access to Bill and Hillary Clinton, yet we seem to know quite a lot about their public and private lives, and equally there are many people with whom we are in everyday contact whose lives are a closed book to us.

Confidentiality is more specific. It concerns the use we make of information about a person once we have gained, or been given, access to that information. Thus, as Sieber (1992) points out, privacy has to do in the first instance with persons, whereas confidentiality refers to data. Anonymity, meanwhile, concerns not access to information, nor its disclosure, but its assignment or attribution to specified individuals. Figure 5.1 illustrates the concepts of privacy and confidentiality in relation to client information.

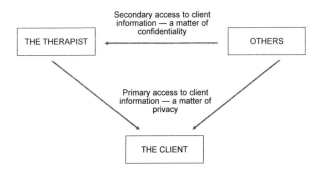

Figure 5.1 The relationship between privacy, confidentiality and client information

It should also be noted that one's privacy is distinct from one's sense of privacy (Beauchamp and Childress, 1994). A person's privacy may be invaded without his or her knowledge, leaving the person's sense of privacy intact. Conversely, attempts by others to gain information about a person may be fruitless, but may nonetheless give rise to a feeling of loss of privacy.

The circle of confidentiality

In their discussion of this topic, Brown *et al.* (1992) introduce the helpful concept of a 'circle of confidentiality'. This circle, which will vary in size in different situations, consists of those people with whom confidential information can legitimately be shared. On very personal matters, the circle may consist of just one or two people, whereas in other cases it may extend to a large number.

In the context of multidisciplinary health care, it may be necessary to share information with a number of team members in order to care for the patient safely and effectively. On the receipt of confidential information from another person, one is given entry to the circle as one might be admitted to membership of a club. However, just as in the case of club membership, the person introducing others to the circle must ensure that they are aware of the rules, i.e. that the information is privileged and that certain criteria govern its disclosure. The therapist must therefore think carefully before admitting other people to the circle; the key question is 'do they need to know'? For many items of information, it can be argued that other health professionals closely engaged in the patient's care do need to know, whereas colleagues who are only tangentially involved with the patient, or who are merely displaying a professional interest in the patient's condition, do not. There are other situations in which the sharing of information may have even less in the way of justification; what Siegler (1991:183) calls 'the wanton, often inadvertent, but avoidable exchanges of confidential information that occur frequently in hospital rooms, elevators, cafeterias, doctors' offices, and at cocktail parties'.

Downie and Calman (1994) suggest that, when considering potential recipients of information, these individuals should be separated into four groups: (1) those who must know; (2) those who should know; (3) those who could know; (4) those who shouldn't know. In this way, therapists can gauge the permissibility of communicating privileged information in terms of the recipient's relative need to be acquainted with it. Categories 1 and 4 are of course clear-cut, whereas categories 2 and 3 may give rise to some uncertainty.

Of course, the patient is also entitled to control access to the circle – more so, perhaps, than the therapist. We shall see shortly the problems that may arise if patient and therapist operate different criteria for admission.

Because other individuals than the patient can provide entry to the circle of confidentiality, it follows that there need be no direct contact, and therefore no specific prior agreement, between patient and therapist for a duty of confidentiality to exist. Indeed, questions of confidentiality may arise in relation to information of which the patient is unaware, such as when a doctor breaches confidentiality by disclosing a diagnosis to a third party before it has even been communicated to the patient. Hence, Gillon is not strictly correct to assert that 'there can be no transgression of confidentiality if the information is not regarded as secret by the person giving it' (Gillon, 1986:108). Even where there is direct contact, there need be no specific demand for confidentiality from the patient, nor an explicit pledge on the part of the therapist. If the therapist comes into the possession of information indirectly or by chance, the requirement to maintain confidentiality arises just as it does when such information is specifically entrusted. As Kottow (1986:119) points out: 'Information fortuitously gained within the freely chosen association of the clinical encounter is to be considered confidential and treated in the same way as information voluntarily disclosed by the patient'. The therapist should consider carefully the nature of the information disclosed:

> Mary Eames has anorexia nervosa. During an emotional moment in a counselling session, she tells her occupational therapist, Joy Rogers, that she attributes her present feelings about her body to a series of unsuccessful sexual encounters earlier in her teens.

Here, the requirement to keep such information confidential stems not from any explicit request from Mary, nor from specific assurance on Joy's part, but from the implicit understanding that such matters to do with a person's sexuality are regarded as sensitive and a potential cause of embarrassment. However, it is fair to say that where there is a specific request from the patient, and/or a specific assurance from the therapist, this adds extra weight to the duty of confidentiality.

Nonetheless, confidentiality may still not be absolutely binding, for it may be that the notion of confidentiality contains within it a certain latitude, to cope with serious and unexpected contingencies. The analogy with promising is relevant here:

> The institution of promising has built into it an element of discretion and vagueness over the bindingness of most types of promise, and we have good reason to preserve this feature of promise-making: we both want to tie people to act as agreed, and not to tie them too tightly, since neither we nor they can foretell precisely what will happen and what may turn out to be desirable. (Jackson, 1994:490)

If confidentiality is not absolute, there will sooner or later be cases in which a conflict between it and some other moral imperative must be resolved. However, before considering specific practical issues to do with privacy and confidentiality, it is necessary to explore these concepts and their moral origins more fully.

The grounds of privacy and confidentiality

Privacy has a firm foundation in the principle of respect for autonomy. Autonomy has to do with controlling one's life for oneself, and this includes control over information about oneself. Access to a person is only legitimate, it can be argued, if such access has been autonomously authorized by that person. Furthermore, an individual's plans and projects may depend for their success on what others know about his or her intentions.

However, to ground privacy solely in autonomy is perhaps to provide an incomplete defence of privacy. In particular, it suggests that those who cannot exercise autonomy have no right to privacy. Hence it is useful to import the allied principle of respect for persons to give additional support to the right to privacy. A person who is comatose or severely mentally ill may not be capable of autonomous action, but may still possess an essential dignity as a human being which would be undermined by a breach of privacy.

Maintaining confidentiality, like privacy, derives support from the principle of respect for autonomy. This is demonstrated by the fact that one can autonomously agree to the divulgence of confidential information. On many occasions, however, it is also supported by considerations of non-maleficence. Information is not revealed to others because, if it were known, it might bring about harmful consequences for the person concerned. Thus, the principles of respect for autonomy, respect for persons and non-maleficence provide a moral basis for privacy and confidentiality. On the basis of such principles, there is a *general* duty of confidentiality towards everybody with whom we come into contact. In addition, a *specific* duty of confidentiality can be identified in the patient–therapist relationship. This has much to do with the exercise of power within this relationship. As Bok indicates, the possession and control of information, by oneself or others, affects the balance of power in human relationships:

> To be able to hold back information about oneself or to channel it and thus influence how one is seen by others gives power; so does the capacity to penetrate similar defenses and strategies when used by others. (Bok, 1984:19)

Thus, when a patient gives personal information to a therapist this is a transfer of power. The professional is given access to information to which he or she would not normally be privy, and the patient is potentially vulnerable to the use that the therapist may make of such information. However, there is an implicit condition attached to such access: the information is not to be used in ways that will harm the patient. Thus, in surrendering some measure of personal privacy, the patient grants the therapist right of access, but in the process the therapist incurs a duty of confidentiality.

Furthermore, it is important that the power gained by the therapist through the possession of confidential information is not misused for purposes of self-aggrandizement, to promote inter-professional rivalries, or to establish professional territories. Hart and Bond (1995) provide an example of the last of these in their account of an action research project in a residential institution for elderly people. In order to understand the health-related needs of a resident, the staff contacted her general practitioner (GP):

> Although Miss A readily agreed to allow the manager to ask her GP to enlighten them both about her health so that staff could better meet her needs, the doctor was enraged by this request. He wrote across the home's medical records in large red print, 'Diagnosis is a confidential matter between doctor and patient' and then threatened to make a complaint to the local authority about the incident. (Hart and Bond, 1995:171)

The authors go on to draw attention to the way in which 'the medical ethics of clinical judgement and clinical confidentiality may be invoked in a manner which thwarts staff's attempts to act responsibly' (Hart and Bond, 1995:174).

Moral conflicts associated with confidentiality

We have seen that the therapist has both a general and a specific duty of confidentiality. However, as with the duty of veracity, this is a prima facie, not an absolute, duty. It may, and often does, come into conflict with other duties which the therapist is required to observe. Consider the following examples:

> A physiotherapist is treating a young woman, Marie Davis, for a haematoma on her arm. During treatment Marie becomes tearful and admits that the injury is the result of her husband hitting her in a fit of temper. Grateful for somebody to talk to, she tells of problems at home, and comments 'It's not really me I worry about, it's when he hits the kids that I get frightened'. She insists, however, that this must go no further.

> Following a flexor tendon repair, James Preston, a telephone engineer, is attending the occupational therapy workshop. On the day in question, he suddenly has an epileptic fit. When the fit subsides a few minutes later, the patient reveals to the therapist, Janine Scott, that nobody has ever witnessed one of his fits before, and nobody else is aware that he is prone to them. Knowing that the patient drives a car as part of his work, the therapist urges him to speak to his family doctor about his fits. He refuses to do so.

> A physiotherapist is treating Mary Sorrell, a middle-aged woman referred by her family doctor for a frozen shoulder. While examining the joint,

the therapist, Siân Allen, notices swelling in the axilla around the pectoralis major muscle and a puckering of the skin over the lateral aspect of her breast. On questioning Mrs Sorrell about this, Siân learns that she has found a lump in her breast. She ask Mrs Sorrell whether she has seen her doctor about this, but she says that she hasn't, and will not do so as her mother underwent a radical mastectomy at her age and she does not wish to undergo the same experience. Siân cannot persuade her to change her mind on this.

The first two cases illustrate the most common conflict to occur with respect to confidentiality; that between the duty to preserve the confidentiality of information and the duty, based on beneficence, to protect others from danger. The latter is often advanced as a possible justification for a breach of confidentiality:

> Any decision to break confidentiality must be clearly justified; in most instances, except when a distinct harm would be prevented, this act is extremely difficult to justify. (Fromer 1981:337)

Our immediate response, perhaps, is to say that the duty to prevent harm should indeed override the duty of confidentiality. This would certainly seem to be a reasonable consequentialist reading of the situation; the harm to others which may be caused by maintaining confidentiality is apparently far greater than that which the patient is likely to suffer if confidentiality is breached. Not everybody would agree with such a conclusion, however.

One objection to disclosure might refer to the very nature of confidentiality, and argue that if the duty of confidentiality is allowed to yield to considerations of utility, it becomes largely meaningless. From this deontological perspective, a pledge of confidentiality is, by definition, to give an assurance that information will be withheld from others even when it would seem that a better outcome overall would come about through revealing it. As Ellos (1990:3) points out, 'confidentiality is concerned not with the greatest good of the greatest number but with the individual good of the patient'. If an assurance of confidentiality meant no more than 'I will keep the secret unless it is better, all things considered, not to do so', this would be to nullify its distinctive nature as an assurance. Warnock demonstrates this in his discussion of the problems of grounding the promises made by a doctor purely in notions of utility:

Though he might, if I asked him, promise not to kill me off, he would of course keep this promise only if he judged it best on the whole to do so; knowing *that*, I could not unquestioningly rely on his keeping it; and knowing that, he would realize that, since I would not do so, it would matter that much less if he did not keep it. And so on, until his 'promise' becomes perfectly idle. (Warnock, 1971:33)

Thus, an argument to the effect that 'where the maintenance of confidentiality results in the moral interests of others being violated, the principle [of confidentiality] can and must be overridden' (Johnstone, 1994:254) would seem, as it stands, to misconstrue the very essence of confidentiality. Does this mean, then, that confidentiality will always be wholly inviolable? Not necessarily, for we have noted that confidentiality is best seen as a prima facie, not an absolute, constraint. However, it should only be breached when the stakes are sufficiently high. It is not enough to argue that better results would accrue by disclosing a piece of information than by withholding it; this only becomes a persuasive argument once a certain threshold is reached. We may legitimately keep confidences, *even if* doing so causes a degree of distress or pain to others, but when matters of life and death are at stake, as they are perhaps in the case of James Preston described above, then the threshold is reached at which confidentiality can be overridden. Thus, while we are not normally obliged to break confidences just because the outcome of so doing is better in consequentialist terms, nonetheless if the results of keeping a confidence are sufficiently dire, we can justifiably reveal information which will avert such an outcome.

Another defence of confidentiality points to the intimate connection which we have identified between confidentiality and the client–therapist relationship. This, it might be argued, gives confidentiality a special status within this relationship, to the extent that to undermine confidentiality is to destroy the essence of this relationship. This justifies health professionals in placing confidentiality to their patients above the interests of others with whom they have no special relationship (Kottow, 1986). Thus, through this relationship, Janine Scott has a responsibility to James Preston which she does not have to other members of society who may be endangered when he is driving his car.

Whether one accepts such an argument depends upon one's view of the moral status of the professional role. If this role gives responsibility to the individual patient or client a specific priority over responsibility to society at large, then confidentiality will enjoy a privileged position. Conversely, if duties to the individual are seen as more on a par with duties to society, then confidentiality is in some cases liable to be subordinated to the 'greater good'. The balance here may differ between professions in terms of their perceived roles. While it would be dangerous to make broad generalizations, a medical social worker might feel a greater professional responsibility for the welfare of Marie Davis's children than a speech and language therapist, though it is not clear that there would be such a difference with respect to the other road-users whom James Preston might harm.

Finally, a defence of confidentiality can be mounted in consequentialist terms. Confidentiality should be respected not because it is by definition an intrinsic part of the therapeutic relationship, but because it is instrumental to the success of therapeutic activities (Walters, 1978). Unless patients can reliably depend upon the discretion of those who care for them, they will be reluctant to disclose potentially sensitive or damaging information. Such information is frequently vital to the process of assessment and subsequent treatment planning, and without it the prospects of a successful clinical outcome are remote. This is particularly the case in psychiatry, where the disclosure of thoughts or experiences which are stigmatizing or potentially damaging to the client is often a vital part of the therapeutic process. Furthermore, even if the disclosure of confidential information on a particular occasion might seem to have beneficial consequences, in the long term such a practice on the part of health professionals would be counterproductive. If information about patients' epilepsy, HIV status, thoughts of self-harm, and the like, is not to be regarded as privileged, patients will in due course no longer seek help for such problems in the first place (Kottow, 1994).

A consequentialist argument can also point to the *likelihood* of the harm which may accrue if confidentiality is either maintained or relaxed. Koehn (1994) and Kottow (1986) both point out that the harm to the patient in breaches of confidentiality is definite, whereas the harm to others if confidentiality is kept is usually only probable.

So far we have been considering breaches of confidentiality for the good of others. However, the case of Mrs Sorrell illustrates a situation in which a health professional might wish to breach confidentiality for the good of the patient. Similarly, in the cases of Marie Davis and James Preston, it is not just the interests of others that are at stake. Can there be a justification for paternalistic breaches of confidentiality? The first thing to note is that in the cases above such paternalism must necessarily be 'strong' in terms of the distinction outlined in Chapter 3, as a specific desire for confidentiality has been voiced by the patient. In any case, to argue that overriding confidentiality is in the interests of the patient is to engage in a logically suspect piece of reasoning. Surely one of the individual's key interests is to have his or her autonomy respected, and it is precisely this that is threatened by a breach of confidentiality. It is unlikely, therefore, that disregarding the patient's wishes will be deemed morally acceptable in such cases, unless evidence can be put forward to suggest that the patient is in some way incompetent.

However, there is another relatively common situation which may be less easy to resolve. This is where information about a patient's condition is revealed to members of the family, prior to any disclosure to the patient him- or herself. The reason for doing this is often to determine whether the patient would wish to know, or to establish the best way in which to break the news; as such, the paternalism involved could be said to be 'weak'. Nonetheless, in the light of the arguments favouring truthfulness discussed in Chapter 3, such abrogation of confidentiality would rarely be justifiable. The lack of full respect for patient autonomy in such cases of concealment, compounded by the breach of confidentiality, would tend to outweigh the intended beneficence of the action.

Finally, it should be noted that confidentiality is an example of an issue on which legal and ethical demands may differ quite radically. The due process of law may demand that confidential information be disclosed, 'in the public interest', in situations where the health professional would very likely feel it morally wrong to do so. It should be remembered that information shared between patient and health professional has no privileged status in UK law, in the way that it does between lawyer and client. Equally, the practitioner may on occasions feel morally impelled to reveal information where doing so could bring a civil action for negligence (Brazier, 1992).

Conclusion

The issue of confidentiality arises for therapists in all sorts of everyday situations. The basic presumption should clearly be that all information relating to clients should be treated as privileged, and that the circle of confidentiality should be guarded conscientiously. However, cases will arise in which there are arguments favouring the disclosure of privileged information. The permissibility of breaching confidentiality should be carefully considered, but a decision to do so should only be taken when the harm likely to be caused by maintaining confidentiality is sufficiently serious. In particular, a consequentialist line of reasoning which makes confidential information vulnerable to calculations of marginal benefit is misguided, as it denies the very essence of confidentiality.

The question of confidentiality with respect to HIV infection will be considered in Chapter 9.

6

Death and dying

It might at first seem rather strange to include the topic of death and dying in a book aimed at therapists. After all, while therapists often come into contact with patients who are at or near the point of death (McAteer, 1997), they do not usually take the decision to end a patient's life or to withdraw life-sustaining treatment. Nor do the techniques and modalities employed by therapists often have the potential either to save or to terminate a patient's life. However, this topic is of very real relevance to therapists, and merits careful consideration. This is for three principal reasons:

1   Although they may not *initiate* a decision to discontinue active treatment, therapists are generally expected to *participate* in such a decision. Whether they like it or not, therapists are often intimately involved in the carrying through of such decisions (e.g. the issue of 'do not resuscitate' orders, to be considered later).
2   Similarly, even though they may not be the prime movers in decisions affecting the life and death of a patient, therapists may be able to influence such decisions if, for example, they are taken in the context of a meeting of the multidisciplinary care team. Alternatively, therapists may find themselves sitting on committees which have an *influence* on institutional policy towards euthanasia or the implementation of life-saving treatment (e.g. a therapist might be a member of a hospital ethics committee charged with formulating or approving such a policy).
3   Even if the preceding points are not thought convincing, and it is felt that matters of life and death do not impinge

significantly on professional practice in the therapies, it can still be argued that therapists should take an active interest in ethical questions that affect other spheres of health care, beyond the immediate confines of their own professional activities.

The ethical issues addressed in this chapter will primarily be those connected with the termination of life. Although some of the ethical issues to do with terminal care will be touched upon in passing, these will not be a primary focus of this chapter. The question of suicide will be addressed in Chapter 9.

Euthanasia

Etymologically, euthanasia comes from the Greek, and literally means 'a good death'. There are in fact two senses in which such a death should be good: it should be good in terms of how it occurs, and it should occur for reasons that are morally good. The second question is perhaps the harder to resolve – it is perhaps easier to agree on the best way in which death should occur (e.g. swiftly, painlessly and in a dignified manner), but when and why it should occur can give rise to difficult conflicts.

At this point, it is important to clarify some definitions. In a case of euthanasia, killing is performed by the action, or inaction, of somebody else; if somebody aids a patient in killing himself or herself, this is known as assisted suicide. According to McLean and Maher (1983), there are three types of euthanasia:

1 *Voluntary euthanasia.* This occurs when a patient, with the capacity to decide, requests, or agrees to, the termination of life.
2 *Involuntary euthanasia.* This occurs when either of the following apply: (a) the patient has the capacity to decide but has not been consulted; (b) the patient has the capacity to decide and has declined euthanasia.
3 *Non-voluntary euthanasia.* This is euthanasia in a case where the patient cannot decide for one of two reasons: (a) the patient has lost the capacity to decide, e.g. through coma or acute mental illness; (b) the patient has not developed the

capacity to decide, e.g. children, those with severe learning difficulties.

In some cases of apparently non-voluntary euthanasia, action may be taken on the basis of an 'advance directive' previously drawn up by the patient concerned. The function of an advance directive is as follows:

> Advance directives are documents which set out in advance of incompetence, through ageing, accident or disease, how a person wishes to be treated. (Fletcher *et al.*, 1995:220)

An advance directive may take the form of a *living will*, in which the patient specifies those treatments or procedures he or she would wish either to receive or not to receive in the event of incompetence, or a *durable power of attorney*, which is a document empowering another person to make decisions on behalf of the signatory (Beauchamp and Childress, 1994). The two varieties of advance directive may, of course, be complementary, with the person nominated under a power of attorney being given the responsibility of discharging the provisions of a living will (Brazier, 1992). In such situations, because death is in accordance with the individual's prior expressed wishes, an argument can be made that this is really a case of voluntary euthanasia.

The moral implications of these forms of euthanasia will be considered in turn.

Voluntary euthanasia

The key moral concept at stake with respect to voluntary euthanasia is autonomy. To permit voluntary euthanasia would seem to be an obvious act of respect for the patient's autonomy; the right to self-determination should include the right to self-termination, as it were. Indeed, it might be argued that respect for the patient's autonomous wishes does not just make it morally *permissible* to engage in voluntary euthanasia, it may even make it morally *obligatory* to do so. There are, however, a number of objections to voluntary euthanasia, six of which will now be considered.

1   The first such objection concerns the scope of autonomy. It might be argued that although individuals should have autonomy *within* their lives, this does not imply autonomy *over* their lives. Many Catholics take such a view, arguing that our lives are not ours to dispose of as we wish; life is a 'gift from God', but it is one over which we do not have absolute ownership, but a form of stewardship. Similarly, within Protestantism, suicide and voluntary euthanasia may be seen as a contravention of the sixth commandment, 'do not kill' (Trowell, 1973). It is important to note, however, that arguments such as these will presumably also tend to rule out all other forms of killing, as there is no logical reason why they should apply only to cases of suicide or killing at the request of the 'victim'. Indeed, if we are not permitted to take our own lives, it would seem to be even more the case that we shouldn't take the lives of others. However, many of us feel that killing may be justified in some instances – in self-defence, for example, or in the course of a just war. In such cases there are, presumably, good reasons which override the usual prohibition against killing, and there might be equally good reasons in the case of suicide or euthanasia. A prohibition against killing would seem to operate much more forcefully against the involuntary ending of life, by whatever means, than against voluntary euthanasia.

2   A second problem raised with voluntary euthanasia is that of deciding whether the request is indeed an autonomous one. Perhaps patients in great pain or distress are unable to form truly autonomous requests – we have already noted in Chapter 4 that this can be hard to judge. Another sense in which such a request may be less than autonomous is if patients feel the need not to be a 'burden' to others. Friends, relatives or health professionals may convey such an impression to patients, albeit not always intentionally. There are also practical problems with determining the autonomous nature of a request for euthanasia. In some cases, the problem may relate not so much to the underlying autonomy of the patient's wishes, but to the expression of such wishes. Especially in cases of impaired communication (e.g. ventilator-dependent patients, or those on high doses of pain-killing

medication), the request for euthanasia may be ambiguous; can we be absolutely sure that an apparent request to die is what it seems? Great care must obviously be taken to gain an unequivocal expression of the individual's wishes.

This objection has some force to it, but it would not seem to be an objection to voluntary euthanasia in principle. Rather, it is an argument for devising valid procedures for determining the competence of potential candidates for euthanasia, and building in the necessary safeguards.

3   Even if there are no doubts as to the autonomy of the desire for voluntary euthanasia, some critics of this practice raise a third objection. They deny that it should be permitted on the grounds that it is likely to be the thin end of the wedge, or the first step on a 'slippery slope'; once it is permissible to kill somebody under these circumstances, it may prove impossible, or at least very hard, to prevent this occurring in other circumstances where it would not be justified.

Lamb (1988) indicates that such slippery slope objections can take two forms. The 'empirical' form claims that an acceptance of voluntary euthanasia is likely, as matter of fact or probability, to lead to future abuses; a practice established for merciful reasons may be hijacked by those whose motives are essentially merciless. The 'logical' objection makes a somewhat different point. It argues that, once the prohibition against killing has been relaxed, it may not be possible to maintain firm logical or conceptual distinctions between practices of killing which are morally acceptable and those which are not. Here, Lamb points to the possibility that euthanasia which is authorized in respect of those who are a nuisance to *themselves* may be extended to those who are a nuisance to *others*. He argues:

> It is very hard to maintain a clear distinction between judging the uselessness of one's own life and someone else's judgment regarding the uselessness of the life in question. In a very important sense our opinions of ourselves are often grounded on the opinions of others. (Lamb, 1988:65)

The force of the slippery slope argument is not, therefore, that there is necessarily anything wrong with voluntary euthanasia itself, but that it may be the source of other practices which *are* wrong.

Other writers, however, reject the use of the slippery slope principle. Rachels argues that one can find a clear basis for separating acceptable and unacceptable cases of euthanasia:

> There *are* rational grounds for distinguishing between the man in agony who wants to die and other cases, such as that of an old infirm person who does not want to die. It is easy to say what the rational ground is. It is simply that in the first case the person requests death, while in the second case the person does not request it. (Rachels, 1986:173)

Notice also that the potential confusion which Lamb pointed to between being a nuisance to oneself and being a nuisance to others was one relating to *why* a person might want to die. This is not the same as identifying a confusion as to *whether or not* a person wishes to die, and as long as this latter distinction can reliably be established, the slippery slope argument loses its bite.

Another riposte to the idea of the slippery slope is made by Harris (1985). He emphasizes the fact that the initial step onto the slope is not intrinsically wrong, and that problems only arise with subsequent downwards movement towards an unacceptable conclusion. He further argues that slippery slopes are only dangerous 'if they catch us unawares and we have strayed onto them inadequately equipped' (Harris, 1985:127). The fact that performing an action now that is right *may* lead us subsequently to do something wrong is not necessarily an argument against doing the initial action. As Harris comments, in reference to in vitro fertilization:

> It would be irrationally self-defeating if we decline to permit work which is in no way immoral and which can benefit us all, merely because we fear that at some future time we will not have the courage to object to work that *is* immoral. (Harris, 1985:127)

It is doubtful, therefore, that the slippery slope argument is strong enough to rule out voluntary euthanasia. It serves more to underline the stringent safeguards that must be built into any policy of assisted death.

4   A fourth criticism of voluntary euthanasia is focused more directly on the role of the health professional. It may be that one should not be party to the taking of life even if it is what the individual desires. Some actions are perhaps intrinsically wrong, and health professionals should not be expected to carry them out, even if they would seem to be morally appropriate in other respects. Furthermore, it might be argued that the taking of life is fundamentally incompatible with the essence of the health professional's caring role.

The first thing to note about this line of reasoning is that it relates more to the suggestion that health professionals should somehow be compelled to carry out euthanasia, not to the notion of euthanasia as such. Providing that there is scope for individual doctors or therapists to exercise conscientious objection, as nurses may in relation to abortion, and assuming that another practitioner with no such objection can be identified, this argument does not preclude voluntary euthanasia from taking place. Second, this point of view smacks rather of what has been called 'moral self-indulgence' (Williams, 1976); the desire to 'keep one's hands clean' by not performing distasteful actions oneself, even at the cost of failing to attain a morally desirable goal. Finally, as will be suggested shortly, it is debatable whether performing voluntary euthanasia is necessarily an 'uncaring' thing to do.

5   A fifth counter-argument to voluntary euthanasia is that, once the practice is accepted, this will remove the impetus behind attempts to find better means of pain control in terminal care. Our efforts would be better directed towards improving terminal care, so that euthanasia would become largely unnecessary. This is broadly the view of Dame Cicely Saunders, generally regarded as the founder of the modern hospice movement. In support of this view, she has suggested, in a television broadcast, that allegedly lower standards of pain management in terminal care in the Netherlands are linked to the availability of voluntary euthanasia there. When assessing this point of view, we should first of all remember that voluntary euthanasia is not only sought by those in pain. Individuals may feel that their lives are no longer worth living because of severe incapacity

or a profound and irremediable loss of dignity. A person with tetraplegia, severe multiple sclerosis or motor neuron disease may have such feelings, and yet not suffer from significant degrees of pain. Indeed, a recent study of the attitudes of oncology patients found that depression was more strongly associated with a wish for euthanasia or physician-assisted suicide than was pain (Emanuel *et al.*, 1996). In addition to this, Cicely Saunders' point of view shares with the slippery slope argument a certain defeatism. It might be argued that we could allow voluntary euthanasia, and then take the necessary steps to ensure that research into terminal care continues vigorously. It is not inevitable that permitting the former will weaken our efforts in respect of the latter.

In any case, to say that advances in terminal care may make euthanasia unnecessary in the *future* does not settle the question for the *present*. Kasting (1994) argues that pain relief in terminal illness is not yet universally effective; the best we can claim is that the majority of such pain can be relieved. Consequently, the possibility remains that euthanasia is indeed necessary in cases where pain cannot be abolished:

> [W]hen the nonnecessity argument is grounded on the premise that most pain in terminal illness is relievable, the *most* one may conclude is that euthanasia and physician-assisted suicide are unnecessary in those cases where pain and suffering *are* relievable. (Kasting, 1994:25)

6   The final objection to voluntary euthanasia to be considered takes the following form. If doctors are permitted to kill patients, even under carefully regulated conditions and with due attention to the competence of patients and the autonomy of their choices, this will nonetheless irretrievably undermine the trust on which the doctor–patient relationship depends. As one writer has put it:

> [P]utting physicians into the role of executioners would have a potentially corrosive effect on their usual relations with patients. I never want to have to wonder whether the physician coming into my hospital room is wearing the white coat (or the green scrubs) of a healer – concerned only to relieve my pain and restore me to health – or the black hood of the executioner. Trust between patient and physician

is simply too important and too fragile to be subjected to this unnecessary strain. (Capron, 1986:144)

Again, the force of this objection is not really against voluntary euthanasia in principle. It relates more to the way in which euthanasia is presented, and to possible abuses of it. If the process is seen as cold, dispassionate and to a degree ruthless, it may well be the case that patients will come to be fearful and distrusting of doctors. However, it need not be so. Recently, a case of voluntary euthanasia in the Netherlands was recorded as it occurred, and broadcast on UK television. The overwhelming impression that this left on many people was that euthanasia can be a supremely compassionate and caring action on the part of a medical practitioner. Indeed, portrayed in this way, euthanasia may serve to increase a particular form of trust in the doctor–patient relationship – a trust in the doctor's ability and willingness to perform the action that is likely to be the last resort for those who otherwise have no hope of relief from an intolerable situation.

A number of objections to voluntary euthanasia have been examined. Each has been shown to have shortcomings, and it is doubtful that any has sufficient weight to overturn the powerful autonomy-based presumption in favour of voluntary euthanasia. The question remains, however, as to whether other forms of euthanasia can be justified.

Involuntary and non-voluntary euthanasia

It is hard to think of any possible moral justification for involuntary euthanasia. The only possible way to defend the practice would be to point to the interests of others; to argue, in effect, that while it might be against the interests of the individual to be killed without his or her consent, it might be of benefit to others. The death of a severely disabled elderly woman might, for example, afford an immense relief to those family members responsible for her daily care. Now, while it can be argued on a consequentialist reckoning that certain things can be done to an unwilling individual for the sake of others, including significant restrictions on personal freedom, there are overwhelming arguments to the effect that this must stop well short of an act such as killing. Downie and Telfer illustrate vividly the dangers of such an appeal to the interests of others:

> [M]ight not someone be justified, on this basis, in thinking, 'All right, Granny, you don't want to die. But what's so special about your wants? If it's a matter of wants. we've got force of numbers on our side: I want you to die, and Tom wants you to die, and Dick wants you to die, and Harry wants you to die...' (Downie and Telfer, 1980:45)

With considerations such as this in mind, deontologists point to what they call *constraints* – actions whose intrinsic nature is so morally unacceptable that they are strictly impermissible, even if a great deal of benefit would come about as a result of their performance.

Consequentialists, too, are likely to condemn practices such as involuntary euthanasia, for while superficially it may seem that a net benefit may accrue from it on individual occasions, a broader view reveals that the sort of world that would result from allowing such practices would clearly be worse than one in which they were forbidden. The only circumstances under which one might conceivably justify the killing of an unwilling victim would be to save the lives of a greater number of other people – and even this would be unjustifiable for some philosophers. Moreover, it is hard to imagine circumstances in health care where this would be an issue. Involuntary euthanasia would therefore seem to be unacceptable.

This leaves us with non-voluntary euthanasia. Here, it is hard to see how the principle of respect for autonomy can be appealed to for support, since the individuals concerned are by definition incapable of forming autonomous choices. The closest to this that can be achieved is to argue, on the basis of what one knows about the person concerned, that he or she *would* have wished to die, had the capacity to decide been present. Although this approach has the merit of attempting to remain faithful to the autonomous choices of the individual, it faces the problem that judging such choices will inevitably be an imprecise process, and may be little more than surmise. Of course, if there were pre-existing documentation, such as an advance directive, in which the patient had indicated a desire to die in certain circumstances, there would be no such problem. However, such a case would presumably fall under the category of voluntary euthanasia; non-voluntary euthanasia is, by definition, a situation in which we lack any such clear indication of the individual's true wishes.

An alternative approach to a defence of non-voluntary euthanasia is therefore needed. This might be to claim quite simply that the individual would be better off dead. The appeal here is not to the 'subjective' standard of what this particular person would want, but to the more 'objective' standard of what any rational person would want in the circumstances. Central to this approach is the view that the quality of some forms of existence is so poor that death is preferable. Those supporting non-voluntary euthanasia tend to attach a higher premium to the quality of life than to its quantity; life can have negative value, and there is such thing as the 'good death'. Those against euthanasia, on the other hand, tend to feel that the continuation of life must always be of greater importance than considerations to do with its quality. The underlying conviction is that human life has an intrinsic value that is independent of, and cannot be outweighed by, the quality of the experiences contained within that life. Indeed, Rumbold (1993:81) suggests that the case for euthanasia is inherently confused:

> The question is, if [a patient] is losing his life, his *being*, can this really be said to serve his *well-being*? It is hard to see how a person's quality of life can be improved by the ending of it.

To a large extent, where one stands on this issue will have much to do with one's personal beliefs, which may be religious in their origin, as to the nature and value of human life. However, there are two points which can be made against the critics of non-voluntary euthanasia. In the first instance, it is only correct to suggest that the quality of life cannot be improved by death if one takes a rather literal-minded interpretation of the concepts involved. True, there no longer exists any life of which the quality can be improved, but this is not really the underlying intention; the basic idea is that of removing an intolerable condition, not of substituting it with a better state of being. Second, it must be remembered that in the case of non-voluntary euthanasia, the decisions we take affect not ourselves, but others. Consequently, given that we do not know the specific views of incompetent individuals, we should consider the implications of 'getting it wrong'. There are two alternatives: either we will consign a patient who would have chosen to die to continued pain and distress, or we will end the life of somebody who would rather have continued to live on in suffering. Neither is, of course, a desirable error to make, but it is important not to underestimate the way in which patients have to experience the results of our miscalculation in the first case. Although euthanasia is an irrevocable step, we should consider carefully the alternative of subjecting a person to months of continuing pain and suffering. What at first seems to be the 'safer' option may come at a very great price.

Active and passive euthanasia

Peter Marchant is a 72-year-old man who has just undergone a partial gastrectomy for cancer of the stomach. Although most of the tumour was removed, it was apparent to the surgeon that the peritoneum had been invaded, and there was evidence of metastasis to neighbouring organs. The patient's oncologist is investigating the possibility of palliative therapy, and in the meantime Mr Marchant has been returned to the ward, where he is expected to stay for several days. Following the report of the operation in the patient's case notes, the words 'do not resuscitate' have been written in red ink.

In this case, there is no intention to take positive action to end the patient's life. However, in the event of a cardiac arrest or similar eventuality, it is proposed that no attempt will be made to save the life of Mr Marchant. This illustrates the difference between active and passive euthanasia. The distinction drawn here is between cases in which death is caused by performing a specific action, such as giving a lethal injection (active euthanasia), and those in which death is caused by *not* doing something, such as by withholding treatment (passive euthanasia). Accordingly, active euthanasia is often classed as 'killing' (an act), whereas passive euthanasia is classed as 'letting die' (an omission). Note that whereas the *withholding* of treatment is a case of passive euthanasia, the *withdrawal* of treatment is properly classed as active euthanasia. Therapists are more likely to be involved in passive than in active euthanasia.

There is a strong body of opinion that regards passive euthanasia as less reprehensible than active euthanasia, to the extent that passive euthanasia may be justified in circumstances in which active euthanasia would not. This, presumably, is the view held by the medical team caring for Mr Marchant.

Is there any reason to think that a genuine moral difference exists between these two forms of euthanasia? It is tempting to argue that the apparently greater acceptability of passive euthanasia over active euthanasia is supported by the tendency for the requirement of non-maleficence to be greater than that of beneficence. However, this is not really the case. The distinction in the latter case has to do with the *result* that comes about; it is thought to be worse to bring about a bad result than to fail to produce a good result. Both of these may be the result of either performing or failing to perform particular *actions*. The beneficence/non-maleficence distinction is therefore not really at issue here.

Perhaps, then, the source of the distinction between killing and letting die comes from the fact that in the latter case, but not in the former, one is letting nature 'take its course'. However, it should be remembered that, in the case of Mr Marchant, who has undergone a number of investigations and a major operation, the natural course of events has long since been altered by medical intervention. It is somewhat arbitrary to invoke nature at this particular juncture.

Another argument for the permissibility of passive euthanasia is that, if treatment would be pointless or excessively burdensome for the patient, it is morally permissible to withhold it. However, it makes little sense to talk of the withholding of pointless treatment, because such treatment was presumably never a serious option in the first place. With respect to treatment that is unduly burdensome, the situation is slightly different. Here, purely in terms of therapeutic effect, such treatment is a realistic possibility, but any such therapeutic benefit is deemed to be insignificant in comparison to the harmful side-effects of the treatment. The reason why the benefit of the treatment is insignificant is likely to be because the patient is already near the point of death. However, if this is the case, it is not clear that withholding treatment would play a significant part in causing the patient's death; the question of euthanasia does not really arise. If, on the other hand, the patient is not moribund, but nonetheless it is still felt that life-saving or life-prolonging treatment is too burdensome, the harmful side-effects of the treatment must be very great indeed. In this case, it is once more doubtful that such treatment should be considered as a serious option.

It is not obvious, therefore, that there is a valid moral distinction between active and passive euthanasia. Although there are arguments that can be mounted in its defence (Beauchamp, 1989; Sullivan, 1991), its validity remains a moot issue. In fact, the difference between active and passive euthanasia is more likely to be a psychological or emotional one; in terms of our natural reactions, we may simply find it harder to 'kill' patients than to 'let them die' (Brock, 1989). We may also feel that, by not intervening actively in the patient's death, we have managed to 'keep our hands clean', avoiding some of the responsibility for what has occurred.

Of greater concern is the possibility that the distinction between active and passive euthanasia may lead to decisions on life and death being made on irrelevant and arbitrary grounds (Rachels, 1975). In the case of Mr Marchant, if he experiences a cardiac arrest, he will receive no active treatment and will therefore die. If, however, he does not arrest, he will most likely be discharged from hospital to the care of his family, and will die some time later, or be readmitted for palliative treatment. Which of the two courses of events comes about is determined solely by whether or not Mr Marchant has a cardiac arrest. This is normally a perfectly treatable condition, especially in a hospital environment, and there is no specific indication that the patient would not stand a good chance of making a satisfactory recovery – so why should this be the deciding factor? Presumably the real question is whether Mr Marchant's condition is such that it warrants euthanasia. For this to be decided by the contingency of a heart attack is essentially arbitrary.

More importantly, it can be argued that if there is indeed a moral distinction between acts and omissions in the case of euthanasia, this may be such as to support active rather than passive euthanasia. The conventional distinction between the two varieties of euthanasia is based on the thought that euthanasia is generally undesirable, but that active euthanasia is somehow worse morally than passive euthanasia. However, if it is accepted that in some cases euthanasia is in fact morally justifiable, it would seem preferable to achieve it by active rather than by passive means. If it is thought better not to be actively involved in a bad outcome, by the same sort of reasoning it would seem to be the case that it is better to be actively involved in a good outcome – i.e. just as we should minimize our active involvement in a course of action that is wrong, so we should maximize our active involvement in one that is right: active means are normally a more effective and efficient way of attaining a given outcome than passive means. While active euthanasia may be more distressing for health professionals, it is usually far less painful for a patient who is already suffering than being left to die. Moreover, the factual basis for active euthanasia is sometimes sounder, which may lead to a more informed ethical decision. If we withdraw treatment (active euthanasia), we will have gained first-hand evidence as to the therapeutic effect, or lack of effect, of this treatment, which we would not have acquired if this treatment had been withheld in the first place (i.e. passive euthanasia).

The vital question, therefore, seems to be that of deciding whether or not euthanasia is morally justified in the first place. Whether such euthanasia is active or passive may very well be irrelevant, or if it is relevant, active euthanasia is likely to emerge as the preferable option.

'Do not resuscitate' orders

Quite apart from the question of active versus passive euthanasia, the case of Peter Marchant raises specific issues to do with the policy of issuing 'do not resuscitate' (DNR) or 'not for resuscitation' (NFR) orders. Because a patient may undergo a cardiac arrest in the presence of almost any member of the multidisciplinary team, DNR orders underline clearly the fact that euthanasia is not just a matter for doctors and nurses. Any therapist who works with patients who are, or have recently been, critically ill, or with institutionalized elderly patients, is likely to encounter such orders. The situation may also arise away from the ward: for example, a patient with motor neuron disease, subject to a DNR order, might have a cardiac arrest during a session of speech therapy.

It is important to distinguish at the outset those cases in which a DNR order is instituted because resuscitation is futile and therefore not a viable therapeutic option on technical medical grounds, from those in which resuscitation is feasible, but thought to be ill-advised for various other reasons (Loewy, 1989). In the first case, it is believed that the process of resuscitation simply will not work; in the other case, the process may well work, but this is considered to be a goal not worth pursuing.

It is this latter category that gives rise to the most troubling ethical issues. The first thing to be clear about is that, as the present case illustrates, DNR orders of this second sort are, in nearly all cases, a form of passive euthanasia. Unless a patient is on the very edge of death, or unless resuscitation is deemed medically futile, the effect of a DNR order is to allow a patient to die who would otherwise have a reasonable chance of living longer (even if only for a comparatively short time). It follows from this that DNR orders are not a *clinical* but an *ethical* decision. They rest ultimately upon a moral judgement as to the value of an individual's life. This then prompts the question, on what basis has passive euthanasia been decided upon for the patient concerned? It is vitally important that therapists who are involved in the care of patients subject to DNR orders reassure themselves as to the 'validity' of such orders. There are four key considerations here:

1   If the patient concerned is competent, has the order been instituted with his or her knowledge and consent (Scofield, 1991)? If not, the order is tantamount to involuntary euthanasia, and we have seen that this is unlikely to have any moral justification. Johnstone (1994) suggests that in many cases patients are indeed unaware of DNR orders to which they are subject, especially in residential care for the elderly, where DNR may be the rule rather than the exception. She further suggests that it is inconsistent for residents in such institutions to be asked whether they wish to be cremated, and

where they wish to be buried, but not whether they wish to be resuscitated if the occasion arises. Meanwhile, recent studies suggest that most hospitalized elderly patients do want to participate in decisions concerning the dying process (Kelner, 1995; Bruce-Jones *et al.*, 1996). While it should be acknowledged that consenting to a DNR order may be distressing for patients (Schade and Muslin, 1989), this is not necessarily the case (Bruce-Jones, 1996), and Purtilo warns that 'the decision is such a momentous one that it would take a very strong argument to override the patient's right to be included in this decision' (Purtilo, 1993:163). Loewy (1991) argues that failing to involve patients in such end-of-life decisions is generally an unacceptable form of strong paternalism (as defined in Chapter 3), and is inimical to a process of open communication with the dying patient.

2   Was the order formulated as a consensus decision within the health care team, or unilaterally by a single member of the medical staff? It is surely unfair to ask health professionals to implement such orders if they have had no say in whether they are appropriate in the first instance. Furthermore, the process of discussion within a group will provide an opportunity for the relevant issues to be aired, and if necessary challenged, and will help to prevent decisions being taken on the basis of what might be one individual's flawed reasoning or idiosyncratic views. Therapists often have the opportunity to play an active part in such discussions, and may do much to protect the patient's interests. In particular, by virtue of having more prolonged contact with the patient, therapists may be able to provide insights concerning the patient's hopes, desires and state of mind which are not so readily available to medical staff.

3   When was the order instituted? If a DNR order is not frequently reappraised and updated, we cannot be sure that the factors or circumstances which originally prompted it still apply.

4   Is the order properly documented? Is it totally unequivocal, or is it denoted by a potentially ambiguous symbol or abbreviation (Johnstone, 1994)? Is it absolutely clear to which patient it applies? Has it been clearly signed by its originator? An unsigned order could have been written in the case notes

by anybody, and should on no account be observed until its origin and authenticity has been conclusively verified. In any case, an order that is not clearly attributable is intrinsically suspect. As Johnstone (1994:414) rightly asks, 'if the practice of ordering NFR is so medically, morally and legally justified, why are doctors so reticent in and so loathe [sic] to document their NFR orders formally?'

There is a tendency for DNR orders to be taken at face value, as just one other clinical decision made by doctors in the course of caring for seriously ill patients. Therapists should not overlook the fact that such orders nearly always constitute a form of passive euthanasia and therefore have profound ethical reper-cussions. Moreover, therapists should not underestimate the extent of their involvement in any no-resuscitation policy; at any moment, and without warning, they may find themselves in the position of either implementing the policy or declining to do so. Each of these is an inescapably moral choice, in which the stakes are extremely high.

Case study

To conclude the discussion, a case study will be presented which will highlight some further considerations concerning passive euthanasia that have special relevance to physiotherapists.

> Arabella Dobson is an 84-year-old woman admitted to hospital with bronchopneumonia. She has long suffered from emphysema, and has had several previous admissions for progressively worse acute exacerba-tions of her condition. Mrs Dobson lives alone in a cold, damp ground-floor flat, and is rarely able to go out owing to shortness of breath. Two years ago, she had a cerebrovascular accident, which left her with moderately severe expressive aphasia.
>
> On this occasion she is particularly unwell; she is severely cyanosed, acutely dyspnoeic, and having considerable difficulty expectorating. Antibiotic therapy has been instituted, and intensive physiotherapy is being given in an attempt to clear her chest. It is clear that Mrs Dobson is considerably distressed, and is becoming exhausted by attempts to cough.
>
> Dr Watson-Jones, the attending physician, feels that the patient is in danger of slipping into ultimately fatal respiratory failure, and that,

whatever is done for her, her chances of surviving this episode are probably no more than 50:50. He proposes that Mrs Dobson be given diamorphine hydrochloride to ease her distress and exhaustion, acknowledging that this will suppress her respiratory drive and hasten respiratory failure, and orders that antibiotics should be discontinued. He requests, however, that physiotherapy should be continued as previously.

This hypothetical case study, typical of events that occur in many true-life situations, illustrates a number of problematic issues that arise in connection with euthanasia.

The first of these brings us back to the question of consent. There is no indication that Mrs Dobson has been consulted on the proposed withdrawal of active treatment. Is this reasonable? Although Mrs Dobson is in a state of discomfort and distress, and has moderately severe difficulty in communicating, it is not clear that she is thereby incompetent to participate in decisions regarding her care and treatment. As was argued in Chapter 4, the burden of proof is on the health professional to demonstrate that competence is lacking, not on the patient to demonstrate that it is present. In cases of doubt, competence must be the working assumption, and patients must be consulted. In any case, a judgement as to Mrs Dobson's future quality of life that is not informed by her own preferences and values is fraught with danger in such circumstances.

The second issue that this case raises is the 'doctrine of double effect'. According to this, health professionals can legitimately administer treatment that will ultimately cause the death of a patient, provided that the patient's death is an *unintended* consequence of this treatment. In this way, the prohibition against killing can be deemed not to apply (Beauchamp and Childress, 1994). More specifically, the doctrine requires that:

1   The bad effect (in this case, death) must not be an end in itself, nor a *means* to the good effect (in this case, relief of suffering).
2   The bad effect should be a side-effect, i.e. it is not the objective of the action. The bad effect can be *foreseen*, but it must not be intended.
3   The action itself, independent of its effects, should not be intrinsically wrong.

Thus, it could be argued that the case of Mrs Dobson fulfils these requirements. The objective of withdrawing treatment is not to kill the patient, but merely to ease her distress; although it can indeed be foreseen that Mrs Dobson will die, there is no express intention to end her life. In addition, her death is not the means by which her distress is eased, but is an indirect side-effect of the administration of diamorphine. Finally, in respect of the third criterion, it can be argued that there is nothing intrinsically wrong with the primary action of giving diamorphine to a patient.

There has been much vexed philosophical debate on the doctrine of double effect. Ultimately, whether one finds the doctrine convincing will tend to be determined by the relative importance that one attaches to intentions as opposed to outcomes. Not surprisingly, those whose outlook is primarily consequentialist are hostile to the doctrine (Glover, 1977; Kuhse, 1984; Harris, 1985). A specific weakness of the doctrine is perhaps its reliance on rather fine and philosophically controversial distinctions between consequences that are intended and those that are foreseen but unintended, and between the direct and indirect effects of an action. The possibility exists that health professionals might try to wriggle out of their responsibility for an act of euthanasia by a piece of semantic sleight-of-hand.

The third question which this case prompts it that of 'when is enough enough'? At what point does treatment become harmful rather than beneficial? Jackson (1992) rightly points out that doing more *to* the patient is not the same as doing more *for* the patient. Deciding when to discontinue active treatment is notoriously difficult. One argument which may support cessation is that treatment may reach the point of being unduly burdensome for the patient, such that its harms outweigh its benefits. If an intervention is causing a patient great suffering, and yet is providing insignificant therapeutic benefit, or is prolonging life to a negligible degree, it may be thought that its discontinuation is in the patient's best interests. This requires a careful weighing up of the harms and benefits of the treatment concerned, and wherever possible the patient should participate in this process. In the case of Mrs Dobson, there are reasons to think that, in terms of balancing harms and benefits, it is *not* yet time to discontinue treatment: (a) with a 50:50 chance of surviving her present exacerbation, her prognosis is, by the standards of critical care medicine, quite good; (b) given the nature of her underlying condition, if continued treatment is successful, she has a fairly good chance of regaining her level of functioning prior to this episode.

In conjunction with the balancing of harms and benefits, another factor which may support the withdrawal of treatment has to do with the notion of dignity and the principle of respect for persons. As more and more 'heroic' measures are taken in an attempt to gain an often minor prolongation of life, the patient's personal dignity may be violated. Johnstone (1994) cites the case of a 70-year-old woman being resuscitated 70 times in the course of a few days. It is hard not to think that the preferable course of action would have been to allow the patient to die in a dignified and peaceful manner. Arabella Dobson might in due course reach such a stage, though it is not at all clear that her present condition represents a threat to her personal dignity of sufficient magnitude as to justify euthanasia.

The question of treatment cessation leads us on to the final issue raised by the case of Mrs Dobson. Here, the physiotherapist is placed in the invidious, but not uncommon, position of being asked to continue treatment while other forms of therapy are being withdrawn. It is fundamentally contradictory to discontinue antibiotic therapy and yet request that intensive (as opposed to merely palliative) physiotherapy should continue. This requires the therapist to provide treatment which is likely to be tiring and distressing for the patient, but which has little prospect of producing a therapeutic effect. The motive behind the doctor's request is most probably to be seen to be 'doing something'. Another example of this sort of practice is the use of 'slow codes' for cardiopulmonary resuscitation. Here, resuscitation is initiated in the event of a cardiac arrest, but in a deliberately delayed and half-hearted manner. Again, this is inconsistent. Either it is appropriate to resuscitate the patient or it is not, and if it is, maximum effort should go into the process. Underlying such orders there is usually a misguided attempt by doctors to 'cover themselves' legally and, once more, a desire to give the impression that something has been done. While the appearance of active intervention may possibly give some comfort to the patient's family, it is likely to be psychologically and emotionally distressing to the health professionals involved in the procedure.

For the patient, the procedure is a violation of personal dignity and, moreover, if the resuscitation turns out to be successful, the dilatory manner in which it was performed will increase the chances of brain damage (Purtilo, 1993).

Conclusion

An attempt has been made in this chapter to explore some of the ethical issues surrounding death and dying. Although the question of euthanasia does not present itself to most therapists on an everyday basis, it is a very real issue for those working in acute medical specialties. The fact that the stakes are obviously so high in matters of euthanasia, and that the decision as to whether or not to resuscitate may have to be made without warning, make it all the more important that therapists should clarify their thinking on euthanasia.

7

Resource allocation

This chapter will examine some of the ethical issues which arise in connection with the allocation of health care resources, and will indicate the way in which these impact upon the professional role of the therapist.

Concepts and definitions

For the purposes of this chapter, health care resources can be defined as 'any goods or services that can reasonably be expected to have a positive effect on health' (Buchanan, 1989:293).

It is worth clarifying a few additional definitions at this stage. A distinction is commonly drawn between *macroallocation* and *microallocation*. The dividing line between these two terms is not wholly agreed upon. It has been suggested that macroallocation concerns the nature, quantity and method of distribution of certain goods, whereas microallocation decisions 'determine who will obtain particular scarce resources' (Beauchamp and Childress, 1994:362). Campbell *et al.* (1992:102) argue that macroallocation involves decisions about 'relative spending between types of service provision', while microallocation has to do with 'choices between individuals about who should receive a scarce resource'. Daniels (1985) warns us against drawing too firm a line between these two types of allocation, as they inevitably interact with one another. However, on the basis of the distinctions outlined above, the following definitions can be proposed:

Macroallocation relates to decisions taken in respect of different types of goods or services – either within the health sphere or between this and other spheres – and in respect of certain *categories* of patients. Policies of macroallocation may be formulated by statutory bodies at federal, state, or district level, or by institutions such as insurance companies and other third-party payers (e.g. Medicaid and Blue Shield in the USA).

Microallocation relates to decisions taken in respect of the patient – or of small groups of patients – and usually concerns individual *cases*. Policies of microallocation are likely to arise at the level of a particular institution, unit, or individual therapist.

Finally, there is the notion of *rationing*. While this is sometimes used to describe the distribution of any scarce resource, Caplan proposes a more specific definition: one that 'refers to the distribution of scarce resources that either save lives or significantly enhance the quality of life' (Caplan, 1992:322). Although slightly different interpretations of rationing exist, the term is generally used for a system of allocation that operates under conditions of fairly severe resource constraint.

The right to health care

Underlying most discussions of resource distribution in health care is the question as to whether there is a right to health care. In fact, although there has been considerable debate on this issue (Sade, 1971; Engelhardt, 1991), most people who are happy to talk in terms of rights would agree that such a right does exist. In Chapter 2 it was established that a right of recipience in one person implies a duty of provision on the part of somebody else. Hence, the right to health care entails that there is an obligation on certain members of society – policy makers and health professionals, presumably – to make health care available. The acceptance of a right to health care has clear implications for policies of resource allocation.

A more vexed question concerns the status of such a right. In particular, three subsidiary questions arise:

- Is it a right that we all possess equally?
- Is it a right that we can forfeit?
- Is it a right that can be overridden by other considerations?

These questions will be examined at various points in the remainder of this chapter.

The role of the therapist

It might at first seem that therapists do not play a major role in resource allocation. In terms of macroallocation, this may be true, though therapists should not ignore their capacity to influence policies and decision-making processes through representation on various institutional committees or their membership of professional bodies. It can be further argued that even if therapists do not at present have much to do with macroallocation decisions, in the future they must, willy-nilly, become increasingly involved in this area of activity. Reflecting on the current constraints on health care funding in the USA, Callahan points out the disadvantages that face rehabilitation in competing for funds against other areas of health care:

> Rehabilitation is expensive and resource intensive and does not easily capture public and legislative interest. The outcome of rehabilitation cannot accurately be predicted in each case, and its outcomes have been less well measured than other areas of health care....Most fields of medicine can make a good case for their funding, and some certainly can command a greater sense of urgency and attract public attention more effectively than rehabilitation. (Callahan, 1995:S7–S8)

Therapists ignore issues such as these at their professional peril.

When the focus shifts to microallocation, however, virtually every aspect of the therapist's professional activity, whether clinical or managerial, involves some sort of resource allocation decision. For example:

- Giving appointments for out-patient physiotherapy.
- Deciding which patients on the surgical ward should be listed for weekend treatment.
- Determining the point at which a patient with chronic back pain should be discharged from treatment.
- Deciding whether a patient should be given a custom-made or a cheaper 'off-the-shelf' splint.

- Allocating time during the week for in-service education within a unit or department.
- Deciding which patients should be referred to the domiciliary occupational therapy service on discharge.
- Allocating staff posts between the adult and the paediatric speech and language therapy service within a hospital.

Underlying such examples is the crucial consideration that every action that a therapist takes has what economists call 'opportunity costs'. This simply means that whenever you do something, you could have done something else instead; the cost of performing one activity is the value of the other activities which it has displaced. Hence, every hour spent in a departmental educational programme entails that a certain number of patients are not being treated, and of course vice versa. Resource allocation decisions are thus an inescapable part of everyday clinical and managerial practice.

It is not surprising, therefore, that issues of resource allocation were a major topic of concern for the physical therapists surveyed by Guccione some sixteen years ago (Guccione, 1980). They are likely to be of even greater concern in the present health care climate. In recent years, financial stringency within health care, and specific policies of cost-containment, have brought decisions of resource allocation very much to the fore. In the USA in particular, systems of reimbursement have meant that ability to pay, either directly or indirectly, may be a factor determining the provision of therapy services to individual patients or clients (Cassidy, 1988; Purtilo, 1988; Howard, 1991). Neuhaus (1988) points to the difficulties that may be caused to the therapist by such factors as diagnosis-related groups (DRGs) and the 1982 Health Care Financing Administration ruling in the USA that specifies three hours of therapy a day. She comments:

> It is difficult to set realistic priorities that have some meaning for the patient when the patient's length of hospital stay has been determined on the basis of a diagnostic category that denies the individuality of patients in general as well as the specific needs of that particular person. (Neuhaus, 1988:291)

Therapists have increasingly to work within the context of constraints imposed by third-party payers. This can impede the achievement of desired therapeutic goals, as an occupational therapist interviewed by Gitlin indicates:

> They have 150 days on Medicare. They have to make steady continued progress, and if they don't, they get cut. We have to show documenta-tion that their functional status is getting better, but they are resisting you the whole way. And you want to keep working at it and saying 'Come on and you got to go...' and you give them a few months and then they might do great, but Medicare is going to say they are not cooperat-ing – they're not improving – That's a big problem for me. (Gitlin, 1993:17)

Purtilo and Meier (1995) point out that DRGs do not reflect the complexity of conditions requiring rehabilitation – as a result reimbursement schemes based on DRGs tend to exclude comprehensive rehabilitation. They further indicate that third-party payers may dictate the setting for rehabilitation (i.e. in-patient or out-patient) and the range of treatment that may be provided within it.

It is worth noting that the *Code of Ethics and Professional Conduct for Occupational Therapists* published by the College of Occupational Therapists (COT, 1995) gives detailed guidance on how to deal with the ethical issues resulting from resource deficiency. Meanwhile, the Chartered Society of Physiotherapy has published a detailed Information Paper on the rationing of physiotherapy services (CSP, 1996a). The importance of resource allocation is clearly being acknowledged in professional discourse. Given that decisions on the allocation of resources are an everyday occurrence for therapists, and a source of profes-sional concern, how should they ensure that such decisions are made appropriately? The remainder of this chapter will seek at least partially to answer this question.

Ethical considerations in resource allocation

Broadly speaking, there are three cardinal considerations influ-encing the allocation of health care resources: effectiveness, efficiency and equity (sometimes referred to as the three 'Es'). The first of these is perhaps the most straightforward. It is clearly important that resources are used in such a way that they will

achieve their intended goals. This is supported by a simple application of the principle of beneficence (or, where potentially
harmful interventions are concerned, the principle of non-maleficence).

Efficiency is a more complex issue, as it takes account not only
of the outcome obtained but also of the resources expended in
the process. Thus, two therapeutic approaches might produce
comparable results in the management of a childhood phonolog-
ical disorder, and thus be equally effective, but one of them
might do so more efficiently, such as by producing its results in a
shorter period of time or with less input on the part of the therapist. Again, the underlying principle is one of beneficence: the
more efficiently resources are used, the greater the total benefit
that can be secured.

It is clear that, except for very rare occasions when resources
are not subject to constraint, there must be a concern for
efficiency as well as effectiveness. The very nature of health and
health care requires that the gaining of benefits be balanced
against the expenditure of resources:

> No country is as healthy as it could be and certainly no country can
> afford to do as much for the sick as is currently technically feasible.
> Avoidable death is part of everyday experience. Nor can it be said that
> health is necessarily the most important of competing goals....Given the
> inexactness of need and the almost unlimited scope for the individual to
> consider himself unwell, clearly it is impossible for any society to elimi-
> nate all need. (Cooper, 1975:46)

If, as this quotation suggests, the demand for health care is an
appetite that can never be satiated, efficiency becomes a crucial
moral consideration.

The final consideration, equity, is ethically the most problematic. The notion of equity is broadly equivalent to that of justice
or fairness (Downie and Telfer, 1980). It will be remembered
from Chapter 2 that the principle of justice requires that benefits
and burdens should be apportioned among individuals in a way
that is morally justifiable. Where the benefits concerned are
societal resources, the issues are those of distributive justice.

It might seem that the simplest way to satisfy the requirements
of justice is to distribute resources such that everybody receives
an equal share. However, this takes no account of the fact that

the needs of individuals differ: an equal distribution of resources will produce a very unequal distribution of therapeutic benefit. It would be odd to argue that the patient with residual stiffness of the wrist following a Colles' fracture should receive precisely the same therapeutic input as a patient recovering from severe burns to both upper limbs. Furthermore, there is no specific requirement within the notion of justice simply to treat every-body equally. The criterion is that although one should treat equals equally, one should treat unequals unequally, providing that what makes them unequal is morally relevant; i.e. providing there are morally relevant differences between individuals, it is legitimate to provide them with different levels of therapeutic input. Therefore, to say that everybody has a right to health care is not necessarily to say that everybody has a right to an equal *quantity* of health care.

With this in mind, we can consider some approaches to resource allocation which seek to attain fairness other than simply by giving everybody an equal share. Beauchamp and Childress (1994:330) propose five such alternatives:

1   To each person according to need.
2   To each person according to effort.
3   To each person according to free-market exchanges.
4   To each person according to contribution.
5   To each person according to merit.

These can now be examined in turn, bearing in mind the under-lying need to demonstrate that any inequality of treatment is morally justified.

The first of these approaches seems to be on strong ground, as the respective needs of individual citizens would seem to be a morally relevant basis for allocating health care resources. Furthermore, it is well poised to meet the requirement of efficiency. Given that each person is cared for in relation to his or her needs, there will presumably be minimal over- or under-treat-ment, with the result that resources are not wasted. The technique of *triage*, which is often used in emergency situations, is firmly based on this approach to allocation. Patients are priori-tized for care on the basis of the severity of their remediable clinical need. Thus, those with life-threatening or potentially incapacitating conditions are seen first, whereas those with less urgent problems are required to wait, with the most 'minor' conditions taking their place at the end of the queue. In addition, those who are severely affected by their condition, but for whom little can be done, are given a relatively low priority.

Perhaps the greatest difficulty with this approach to resource allocation is that of distinguishing needs from wants. What one person may see as *necessary* to his or her health and well-being may be regarded by someone else as merely *desirable*. It is hard to arrive at a meaningful distinction between wants and needs, particularly as an argument can usually be produced to show that what seems to be a want is actually a need, and indeed vice versa (Edwards, 1996). Empirical work supports this idea. A procedure such as breast reduction surgery is seen by many as an 'inessential' cosmetic procedure, but a recent study has argued that the operation brings considerable physical, psychological and social benefits, and should be given a higher priority in the allocation of health care funding (Klassen *et al.*, 1996). Nonetheless, although separating what patients want from what they need may be troublesome in some cases, it is often possible to determine the relative need of two or more clients, or groups of clients, with a fair degree of agreement. A crucial consideration is to ensure that assessments of need are informed by the perspectives of clients and patients themselves, and are not unduly influenced by stereotypical or discriminatory value judgements.

What of the second and third approaches? To treat people according to effort is certainly appropriate in some circumstances. We happily pay more to those who work the hardest, and we normally accept that the winner should receive a bigger prize than the runner-up. Moreover, it could be argued that this approach accords with efficiency: those who put the most effort into their health are perhaps the most likely to benefit from the activities of the health care system, just as those who study hardest are likely to benefit most from education. However, its appropriateness to health care has been questioned:

> This is based on the notion of a 'level playing field' on which all have an equal capacity to look after their own interests. However, the reality of ill-health is that it removes the possibility of equality of opportunity in a competitive situation. (Campbell *et al.*, 1992:100)

The very fact of illness or disability disadvantages some people at the outset, and limits their capacity to 'make an effort' comparable to that of the healthy and able-bodied. This is compounded by the major social and environmental barriers that such people face. A system of allocation which ignores this seems particularly inappropriate when these are the people who are most likely to benefit from health care resources.

Much the same objection can be mounted against the third approach. Not everybody is equally equipped to compete in a free-market situation. There are pre-existing differences between individuals in terms of knowledge, skills and financial resources which put some at an advantage over others in the free market. Again, it is not clear that these are morally relevant differences when it comes to distributing a commodity such as health care.

The fourth argument, that health care should be distributed on the basis of social contribution, has a certain plausibility to it. It seems reasonable that the more an individual puts into society, the more he or she should receive from it. Furthermore, it is perhaps equally reasonable that a society should seek especially to safeguard the health of its most productive members, for the ultimate benefit of that society. However, there are difficulties with this position. The first of these has to do with the subjectivity of assessments of social contribution. Who should decide the relative value of different sorts of contribution? Is that of an industrialist necessarily greater than that of a musician or a sanitation worker? It is hard to formulate morally relevant criteria for making such assessments, and even if we could come up with such criteria, it is not clear that the necessary calculations would be reliable, or even feasible. Additionally, there is the familiar 'level playing field' objection. A patient with moderately severe cerebral palsy will have been disadvantaged from the outset in terms of making a contribution to society, however this may be interpreted. Is this a legitimate reason for disadvantaging him or her in the allocation of health care resources? Surely not.

A common everyday situation in which therapists encounter this issue is in allocating appointments for out-patient treatment to patients whose condition has put them off work. These patients are often given some sort of priority, especially in comparison to patients who are not employed, but it is important to be clear why this should be the case. Four possible reasons suggest themselves:

1   The fact that the patient is off work is a reflection of the severity of his or her underlying disability.
2   The patient is suffering an additional disadvantage to that of the condition itself, e.g. through loss of earnings.
3   The patient's dependants are being disadvantaged for similar reasons.
4   The patient is prevented from contributing to society, and has to some extent become a drain on society's resources.

The first reason simply expresses the principle of treating according to need, and does not raise further ethical problems. The second reason would also seem to be morally justifiable. If the therapist can alleviate a greater degree of disadvantage by treating a patient who is off work than by treating one who is not, this would seem to be a morally relevant factor in allocating an early appointment. It should be remembered, however, that not all patients who are off work will necessarily be suffering financial disadvantage, at least initially. The third of the reasons proposed is supported by similar arguments, though it raises the question as to whether the therapist's obligations to a patient's family differ in strength from those to the patient him- or herself.

The final reason is far more problematic. Therapists have to consider carefully the relative weight of their responsibilities to the individual and society in general. It would be a very narrow view which suggested that the therapist only has an obligation to individual patients. It would also be a self-defeating view, because the ability to treat future individual patients will to some degree depend on the general financial welfare of society. Nonetheless, it can be argued that there is a special relationship between therapist and patient which there is not between thera- pist and society, and that this justifies putting the patient's inter- ests first – or at least giving these interests a special weight. On this view, the primary responsibility of the therapist is to serve the needs of patients and clients, not those of society. The fact that the overall benefit produced, in consequentialist terms, might suggest that society's needs should come first is not neces- sarily a conclusive factor. In other words, the patient may be seen as having a right to treatment that should not be overridden by considerations of general social good. We can also imagine the sorts of value judgements that would have to occur if treatment were allocated largely on the basis of the social 'value' of the recipient. Certain sections of society would tend to be discriminated against on what would be, at best, very subjective grounds.

Finally, returning to Beauchamp and Childress's alternatives, there is the argument based on merit. This approach allocates care on the basis not of need, but of desert. This way of thinking accepts that everybody has an equal right to health care, but argues that some citizens may strengthen this right through actions or characteristics which embody personal merit, while others may at least partially forfeit this right for similar reasons.

There is certainly a prima facie acceptability to the idea of treating people according to what they deserve; this, after all, is largely the basis for judicial punishment. However, there are a number of respects in which it is a doubtful basis for the allocation of health care resources. First, it is prone to the problems of subjectivity that were identified in relation to the argument based on social contribution. Second, there is a curious sense in which the notion of desert is backward-looking (Sher, 1987). We might feel that instead of looking at what people have done in the past, we should be looking at their needs at the present and what we can do for them in the future. Third, there is a thin dividing line between a morally legitimate notion of treatment according to merit and a morally illegitimate notion of discrimination. If we were to offer care on the basis of personal merit, we would have to be sure that this dividing line was not being crossed. Fourth, a policy based on desert or merit must accept the fact that some individuals will experience harm, or be denied certain benefits, as a result. Given that there is normally a strong presumption against harming others, or allowing them to be harmed, there is a very firm requirement to demonstrate that this is morally acceptable. Finally, it should be remembered that a policy based on merit does not just mean that some individuals can 'earn' a greater share of health care resources, it also means that other individuals can in various ways disqualify themselves from care and thus, to a greater or lesser degree, forfeit their right to health care resources. These processes are two sides of the same coin, yet many who might find the first acceptable would be uneasy with the second.

In this section, some of the principal theoretical approaches to the just allocation of health care resources have been outlined. Many of these issues will be illustrated in the discussion of some specific issues of resource allocation, to which we will now turn.

Evaluation of health care interventions

It has been stressed that the efficiency of various health care interventions is an important ethical consideration when allocating services. Evaluating efficiency is therefore a crucial activity for health care providers. There are three general approaches to this process, portrayed in Table 7.1. In each case, the cost of an intervention is expressed in monetary terms, but the way in which its outcome is measured differs.

The quality-adjusted life year

Of the above approaches, cost-utility analysis is probably receiving the most serious attention at present (Richardson, 1992). Within this approach, the quality-adjusted life year (QALY) is a radical attempt to provide a mechanism for a comparative evaluation of different treatments or interventions that goes beyond those available within either cost-effectiveness analysis or cost-benefit analysis. The idea of the QALY is to express a health-related outcome in units which represent both the quantity and the quality of that outcome. Hence, while a year of healthy life expectancy would be rated at 1 QALY, a year of relatively unhealthy life expectancy might be rated at 0.6 QALY, or some other figure less than 1. Indeed, a year of life expectancy that was so unhealthy as to be worse than being dead could theoretically be rated at less than 0 QALY (Williams, 1985). The precise ratings of various states of health are generated by surveying the views of the public, asking them, for example, what hypothetical trade-offs they would be prepared to make between the quality of life and its quantity in certain situations. In this way, this form of cost-utility analysis goes further than cost-effectiveness analysis.

Table 7.1 Evaluating efficiency in health care

Approach	Process	Advantages/disadvantages
Cost-effectiveness analysis	Cost of intervention compared to the outcome as expressed in natural units (e.g. increased function, reduced morbidity, reduced incidence of disease)	There is a wide variety of natural units in terms of which outcomes can be measured, but they are not directly comparable with the monetary units of the cost; hence interventions can only be evaluated against alternatives producing the same, or comparable, natural units.
Cost-benefit analysis	Cost of intervention compared to its outcome as expressed in monetary units (e.g. dollars)	The same units are used for the outcome as for its cost, thus facilitating comparison, and permitting an intervention to be evaluated in itself, without reference to alternatives. However, not all aspects of an outcome can be meaningfully expressed in monetary terms.
Cost-utility analysis	Cost of intervention compared to its outcome as expressed in utility units (e.g. QALYs)	Attempts to gauge both the quality and the quantity of an outcome, and hence more comprehensive in its coverage, but it is hard to agree a definition of quality of life. Interventions can only be evaluated against alternatives.

Whereas the latter would seek to measure the number of years added to, or subtracted from, a person's life as a result of an intervention, the QALY approach seeks also to *weight* these years by their quality. For a given intervention, its QALY value is the difference in the number of QALYs with the intervention and the number without the intervention (or with a different intervention).

The use of the QALY is designed to determine one or more of the following:

* Whether a given intervention produces a positive net outcome.
* Which of two or more interventions produces the best outcome.
* Which of two or more treatments is most efficient in producing a given outcome.
* Which of two or more patients will most benefit from a given unit of resource.
* Which types of intervention should be supported by health care resources.
* Which types of public spending, including health care, should be supported by national resources.

Clearly, the QALY can be used for both microallocation and macroallocation decisions. Its originators claim that it has the particular merit of making explicit the sorts of decision-making processes which, they argue, policy makers and health professionals have long been making on the allocation of resources. With a QALY-based system, the assumptions which underlie such decisions are made public, and the process as a whole is open to scrutiny, and thus capable of being challenged.

There are a number of reasons why therapists need to understand the workings of cost-utility mechanisms such as the QALY. Above all, there is the pressure put on therapy services by increasing financial stringency in health care, referred to earlier in this chapter. For reasons which have already been touched upon, the therapy professions may easily find themselves disadvantaged by whatever processes are introduced to reach macroallocation decisions. In addition, even within a set budgetary allocation, there is a need to distribute resources in a way that will prove effective, efficient and equitable. In a similar way, as new interventions and forms of treatment are developed, a systematic means must be found to determine which of these should pass into practice, and which existing treatments should be superseded. The use of the QALY has the merit of highlighting the need to consider the resource implications of all therapeutic decisions.

Widespread use of QALY calculations could also assist therapists in presenting treatment options to patients and clients in a more informative and meaningful way. Dougherty (1994) points out that QALYs can provide patients and their families with a consistent, systematic means of choosing between the benefits of different therapeutic options, and thus potentially enhances the exercise of autonomous choice.

There are, however, a number of ethical difficulties associated with the QALY. The greatest danger is that it threatens to subordinate individual good to collective good, and may thereby sacrifice equity to effectiveness. There are no necessary safeguards within the QALY in terms of a just distribution; a few may be totally neglected for the benefit of the many, or even vice versa, so long as the sums come out right on an aggregate view. Doyal points out that, on the basis of such thinking, 'it would be consistent to argue...that we should allow the 10% of patients who are most sick in all categories to die so that we could use the freed resources more efficiently on the 90% who are less sick!' (Doyal, 1995:274). This reveals the essentially consequentialist basis of the QALY system; it tends to regard individual patients not as individuals, but as sources of QALYs. Indeed, it places no special value on individual *lives*, only on *life-years*. If the saving of one life will produce fewer QALYs than the improving of two or more other lives, the latter should be done in preference to the former if both cannot. This conclusion would be unacceptable to many, and suggests that certain thresholds should be built into any QALY-based allocation system to prevent certain categories of patients from being totally excluded from care. Dougherty comments:

> The immediacy and gravity of some claims can and should overwhelm the abstract generality of QALYs. This is the so-called rule of rescue: the moral obligation to save lives that are in jeopardy. QALY analysis does not capture the moral urgency of these claims. (Dougherty, 1994:64)

Another feature of the QALY system is that it is likely to favour curative interventions over more palliative ones, as the former are likely to have a greater impact on the QALY calculations. This may disadvantage those with chronic, degenerative conditions, many of whom form a large portion of therapists' caseloads. Similarly, the use of QALYs tends to discriminate against those who are already in a poor state of health – their QALY rating is likely to be low to start with – or those who are already close to death, whose potential for generating QALYs is obviously low (Harris, 1987, 1988; Emery and Schneiderman, 1989). This disadvantaging of the ill or disabled is a form of 'double jeopardy':

> [The patient's] first disaster leaves her with a poor quality of life and QALYs then require that in virtue of this she be ruled out as a candidate for life-saving treatment, or at best, that she be given little or no chance of benefiting from what little amelioration her condition admits of. (Harris, 1987:12)

The final objection that can be made to the use of QALYs relates to the basis on which they are calculated. Such calculations are usually based on surveys of the values and opinions of the population at large, the majority of whom are relatively healthy and able-bodied. The outcomes of such an exercise, however, directly affect the minority who are disabled or less than healthy. This raises the question as to whether it is fair to allocate resources to an individual on the basis of general societal values and priorities which he or she may not share? After all, the fact that a life may not seem to be worth living to society at large does not necessarily mean that it is not worth living for the person whose life it is! Able-bodied people often find it hard to appreciate the positive things which disabled people experience within their lives (Morris, 1994). It is important to remember that illness or disability is not necessarily a 'master status'. It is merely one facet of the individual's life, and may have little bearing on the overall quality of his or her life. The disadvantages which are experienced in respect of disability may be more than compensated by positive aspects of the person's social, intellectual or emotional life. Consequently, it must not be assumed that the lives of disabled people are necessarily less rewarding or of lesser quality than those of able-bodied people. In a study of patients with end-stage renal failure, Evans *et al.* (1985) found that individuals' subjective self-assessments of their quality of life were virtually equivalent to those of the general population, despite considerable objective functional limitations. The following statement from a man with amyotrophic lateral sclerosis, which was made via a voice synthesizer, illustrates these point strikingly:

> Throughout the ALS process, I have learned many things. I have learned that ALS does not necessarily mean a death sentence, that I am not living with a life-threatening disease, but rather with a life-enhancing one.
> (cited by Bach and Barnett, 1994:134)

Moreover, quite apart from notions of fairness, it is not clear that the basis of QALY calculation is methodologically valid. It is one thing to determine treatment choices for an individual based on that person's expressed values and preferences, but it is quite another to apply such priorities *across* individuals, each of whom will have different 'scales' of value, with different baselines.

What emerges from this is that the use of the QALY is in tension with the idea of a right to health care. The individual's right to care is subordinate to considerations of overall welfare. It has already been suggested that therapists are accustomed to seeing their work in terms more of caring for individuals than of promoting the good of abstract classes of individuals or of society in general, and they may therefore find this notion hard to accept.

In conclusion, the QALY has a number of merits, but also possesses certain drawbacks when assessed from the point of view of equity. Therapists should therefore exercise caution when using the QALY as a tool for reaching resource allocation decisions.

Where to make the savings?

A problem facing therapists who are confronted with cost containment measures is deciding where within the service to make them:

> An occupational therapy department had a shortage of qualified staff.
> They faced the choice of insisting on giving effective and specific inter-
> vention to a small number of clients or taking the easier path of supply-
> ing a diversional service to a larger number. (Thompson, 1990:135)

In many ways, it is tempting to think that in such circumstances a service – albeit a reduced one – should continue to be
offered to all clients. In this way, any cuts in service are shared by
everybody. After all, it could be seen as discriminatory to
exclude some clients from treatment but not others, and this
would seem to contravene the idea that everybody has a right to
receive care. However, there are problems with this approach. In
the first instance, there is the danger that, while everybody is
receiving *some* care, very few are receiving *adequate* or *effective* care: the jam is being spread so thinly that it can no longer
be tasted! It is also difficult, psychologically and emotionally, to
take on the care of a client, identify his or her needs, but then fail
to address these needs completely. Moreover, this strategy gives
the impression of coping, and may mask the true impact of
resource constraints.

The alternative strategy, in contrast, makes the effect of any
cuts clear to see; administrators, referring medical staff, and the
general public will soon notice if certain clients are excluded
from treatment. It is also likely to be a means of preserving the
overall efficiency of the service. Therapeutic input will be
maintained in those areas where it can accomplish the most
good, and will be withdrawn from those areas in which its effect
is minimal.

On the other hand, there are drawbacks to this approach. As
has been suggested, it runs counter to the idea of a universal
right to care, and may appear discriminatory. More specifically, it
has the disadvantage that whole *categories* of clients will
normally have to be excluded from care. Although it may be
correct to say that a certain group of clients have on average only
minor levels of disability, and thus perhaps only a moderate need
for care, there may nonetheless be some individuals within such
a group whose needs are well above the average. Because these
particular clients will not even receive an initial assessment, they
may be harmed by the lack of care to an unacceptable degree.

In addition, the approach of concentrating resources on certain
clients may not always be the most efficient after all. Very often, a

considerable therapeutic benefit can be achieved in the very early stages of intervention. Even in a single consultation, effective advice on pain-avoidance can be given, self-care strategies can be taught, assistive devices can be prescribed, and an immediate referral to another practitioner can be made when appropriate. Equally, clients may receive considerable psychological benefit from the very fact that somebody has acknowledged and responded sympathetically to their problems, and reassurance from the fact that they have not been totally neglected. Thus, even a limited amount of care may provide a tangible improvement, and even in the face of stringent economies, may be just as cost-effective as a strategy of simply not treating these 'low priority' clients at all.

There is a final problem with cutting some client groups off totally from care. Although, in consequentialist terms, this may seem to be an effective way of highlighting the ill effects of cuts in resources, and of maintaining aggregate levels of effectiveness and efficiency within the service taken as a whole, there is a danger that these individuals will be used solely as a means to an end. This is at variance with the principle of respect for persons outlined in Chapter 2, and as such may be seen as unacceptable by many therapists.

Deciding on a strategy to limit the provision of therapy services is a difficult choice, and there is no clearly right or wrong approach. However, one which excludes certain whole categories of clients would seem to be particularly problematic, and should only be implemented with caution. By way of final comment on this issue, it is worth considering at what level such decisions should be taken. The document *Rationing of Physiotherapy Services* (CSP, 1996a) suggests that physiotherapy managers hold the view that it is the responsibility of the purchasers of a therapy service, not the providers, to decide upon cuts in the service, and to take the consequences of such action. By way of example:

> One purchaser of additional physiotherapy services asked the manager not to treat patients over 65 years old. She insisted that they should make this explicit in the contract with her. (CSP, 1996a:4)

In one sense this is a valid point, but in another sense it is not. As it is the funders of a service, whether these are hospital finance directors or third-party payers, who set the level of resource available to a therapy service, it would indeed seem wrong for them not to be held accountable for the impact of any resulting restriction of service. On the other hand, this does not absolve therapists from the moral requirement to resist what they feel is an unjust policy of resource limitation. Just as 'passing the buck' is unacceptable in the first case, so is a plea of 'just obeying orders' in the second case. The responsibility for resource allocation decisions must ultimately be a shared one.

Conclusion

At the level of both macroallocation and microallocation, there is a need to find a system of allocation that achieves effectiveness, efficiency and equity, without unduly sacrificing any one of these to the others. On the one hand, it is important not to insist of some notion of 'equal therapeutic input for all' if this constitutes a wasteful use of resources. The rights of individuals to receive care should be defined in terms of their needs and the efficient use of communal resources. On the other hand, the goal of efficiency should not be pursued so fervently that certain people are effectively excluded from care altogether. In terms of justice, it may be better to reduce the level of service across the board, so that everybody receives some level of care, than totally to remove some people from care, even if the latter is the more cost-effective strategy. It should be remembered that establishing categories of illness or disability for the purposes of resource allocation can at best be a crude form of classification. A considerable range of need may exist within a particular diagnostic or clinical group, not least because individual clients may react very differently, in psychological terms, to an apparently similar level of 'objective' impairment or disability. Moreover, the basis for decisions to exclude certain categories from care is liable to be morally arbitrary:

> Some illnesses will inevitably be more expensive to treat than others, and sometimes with less effect. Some will not find popularity with the public. Yet neither of these criteria can justify the denial or reduction of health care to those in need. Patients with illnesses which are expensive

to treat or are unpopular can be just as disabled by them as those whose treatments find public favour. (Doyal, 1995:277)

A fair system of resource allocation needs safeguards built into it which will protect those who are especially vulnerable, or particularly powerless to further their own claims and interests. A system which focuses purely on maximizing effectiveness and efficiency – whether through QALY calculations or by other means – will not achieve this. Philosophers such as Rawls (1972) have proposed a different procedure. Societal resources should be distributed in such a way that those who are in the most disadvantaged position are benefited proportionately more – even if this results in an unequal distribution, or submaximal overall benefit for society as a whole. In this way, the interests of justice are allowed to temper the pursuit of efficiency, and the needs of the individual are not wholly subordinated to the needs of the many.

The specific issues surrounding resource allocation to older clients are addressed in Chapter 9.

8

Codes of ethics

It is characteristic of professions in general, and of health professions in particular, that their professional activities are subject to a code of ethics; indeed, possessing a code of ethics is often seen as part of the definition of a profession (Sim, 1985; Purtilo, 1987a; Coates, 1990b). Furthermore, the code can be seen as the creation of the profession, in that the professional body or organization draws up the code, promulgates it, and enforces it.

Codes of ethics in health care are almost as old as medicine itself. The code of Maimonides has been traced back to AD 1135 and the Hippocratic Oath dates from about 400 BC (although it is unlikely that it was the work of Hippocrates himself). An even earlier code has been identified: the code of Hammurabi, dating from about 2500 BC (Guthrie, 1957). The therapy professions cannot claim so time-honoured a pedigree for their codes of ethics. Nonetheless, in 1935 the American Physical Therapy Association (APTA) introduced a *Code of Ethics and Discipline* (Purtilo, 1977); considering the comparative youth of the therapy professions, this was an early initiative. Most national bodies representing the therapy professions now possess a code of ethics of some sort, and codes have also been produced by international bodies such as the World Federation of Occupational Therapists (WFOT).

Functions of the code of ethics

There are a number of manifest functions which a code of ethics may serve. First and foremost, it provides a guide to the practitioner as to conduct which is morally desirable. Hence, the first principle of the *Occupational Therapy Code of Ethics* of the American Occupational Therapy Association (AOTA) states: 'Occupational therapy personnel shall demonstrate a concern for the well-being of the recipients of their services' (AOTA, 1994:1037). Similarly, the corresponding document for speech and language therapists in the UK states: 'The primary professional obligation for all speech therapists is to the long term welfare of their patients' (CST, 1988). In addition, codes of ethics frequently provide guidance on legal matters. Thus, the AOTA code requires members to 'comply with laws... guiding the profession of occupational therapy' (AOTA, 1994:1038), the *Rules of Professional Conduct* of the UK Chartered Society of Physiotherapy (CSP) give detailed advice to members on how to avoid undesirable legal consequences of their actions (CSP, 1996b), and the *Code of Ethics and Professional Conduct for Occupational Therapists* of the College of Occupational Therapists (COT) specifically requires members to adhere to current legislation relating to confidentiality (COT, 1995).

A third function of a professional code is to discourage actions which are unacceptable from a purely professional point of view – those which are not necessarily unethical or illegal, but which are nonetheless undesirable in a professional context. For example:

> Speech therapists must refrain from making laudatory statements about their own personal professional expertise. Any notice or announcement used or displayed must conform to the guidelines issued from time to time by the College. (CST, 1988:2)

> Chartered physiotherapists shall adhere at all times to personal and professional standards which reflect credit on the profession. (CSP, 1996b:2)

As a fourth function, closely linked to the preceding one, a professional code of ethics provides the basis for disciplinary action which may be taken by the professional body against its members (AOTA, 1996). Indeed, the COT document is explicit that the provisions of the code of ethics may be used evidentially for just this purpose (COT, 1995).

Finally, a code of ethics serves as a 'public declaration regarding the societal mission of a group of health care providers'

(Purtilo, 1987a:28). The code is therefore part of the image of itself which the profession seeks to present to the public. Indeed, this notion of declaration is central to the notion of a profession. A profession *professes* certain skills, the use of which is guided by certain values and principles which the profession also professes to hold (Pellegrino, 1979). This notion of a public statement reveals the latent political function of the code of ethics:

> Some commentators argue that codes of ethics are political counters constructed as much to serve as public evidence of professional inten- ℳ tions and ideals as to provide actual behavioural guidelines for practitioners. (Wilding, 1982:77)

The shortcomings of codes of ethics

Despite the fact that codes of ethics are now widespread within the therapy professions, and acknowledging their valuable role in highlighting the need for ethical scrutiny of professional conduct, they have a number of shortcomings. It is worth considering some of these in detail, so as to determine in what ways, and to what extent, codes of ethics can assist therapists in their daily practice.

The code as a consensus view

Because a code of ethics is created by the professional organization on behalf of all practitioners in the particular field, and applies to the profession as a whole, it is often seen as a consensus document. However, this view is subject to two important provisos:

1   The group within a profession that is responsible for drawing up a code of ethics is not necessarily representative of the profession as a whole. Very often, the individuals charged ℳ with creating a code will be senior members of the profession, who may no longer be in clinical practice, and whose values will not necessarily reflect those of more junior practitioners.

2   More crucially, there is no guarantee that those responsible for producing a professional code of conduct represent the values and perspectives of society at large. Veatch (1981) points out that professional ethics are created from within the profession, yet their most significant implications are for those who are outside the profession – patients, clients and their relatives. There is a sense, therefore, in which a code of ethics does not *belong* to those whom it most affects.

The code of ethics will inevitably embody a set of assumptions that spring from a certain perspective on society and morality. Edgar points out that 'assumptions about the authors of the code, the audience, the power relationship between the two, and so forth, will be implicit in any interpretation of the code' (Edgar, 1994:149). Hence, although a code may be framed in very general terms (as will be argued below), the values and perspectives on which it is premised may be very specific, and thus represent a consensus of a very restricted kind.

Such doubts may cause us to question the legitimacy of codes of ethics, particularly as there is rarely any justification given for the particular rules or principles which the codes contain. Speaking of ethical codes in nursing, Singleton and McLaren point out:

> They provide rules for the ethical conduct of a nurse...but there is no indication of what the rationale for these rules might be. What principles are being employed to arrive at these rules? Are they principles with which the nurse, midwife or health visitor would agree? Although these codes clearly provide some level of guidance, without an appreciation of their rationale they cannot be used as a substitute for making ethical decisions. (Singleton and McLaren, 1995:6)

Codes serve several purposes

It has already been noted that codes of ethics have more than one function. The result of this is that their role as a source of specifically *ethical* guidance may be rather obscured. The *Rules of Professional Conduct* of the CSP contain many important statements regarding the rights and welfare of patients (CSP, 1996b). However, they also include advice on the most effective way in which to advertise one's professional services, which seems to have little to do with matters of ethics. Meanwhile, Rule VIII of the CSP code reads: 'Chartered physiotherapists shall adhere at all times to personal and professional standards which reflect credit on the profession'. The concern here is clearly with the interests of the profession, not with those of the patient.

The purpose of individual rules is also unclear. Rule IV reads:

> Chartered physiotherapists shall communicate and co-operate with professional staff and other carers in the interests and with the consent of their patient; and shall avoid criticism of any of them. (CSP, 1996b:2)

The first part of this rule clearly supports the welfare and autonomy of patients, but the second part seems to have much more to do with purely professional matters. Altruistic concern for the patient is merged with issues of professional self-interest.

In a similar way, the first of the *Ethical Principles* of the Australian Physiotherapy Association (APA) is as follows: 'Respect the rights and dignity of all individuals' (APA, 1990:117). This is then analysed in terms of not only the rights of the patient or client, but also the rights of the physiotherapist and those of the profession as a collectivity. In respect of the last of these, it is stated: 'The profession has a right to expect that its good name shall not be brought into disrepute by public argument' (APA, 1990:118).

Again, there is a confusion between genuinely moral concerns and professional self-interest. In both these cases, the possibility is not acknowledged that activities such as engaging in public criticism or argument may, in some cases, actually be a means of furthering patients' interests. This reinforces the earlier suggestion that one of the primary motivating factors for the creation of a code of ethics may be to promote a favourable image of the profession.

The generality of ethical codes

A charge levelled at ethical codes by Singleton and McLaren (1995) is that many of the terms in which they are framed are inadequately defined or explained. One frequently encounters words such as 'rights', 'dignity', 'welfare', 'interests' and 'accountability' used in a rather general way, whereas it was recognized in Chapters 1 and 2 that such concepts need to be used with great clarity and specificity.

Another sense in which codes of ethics may be thought of as excessively general is in relation to the guidance which they give. The exhortation by the Canadian Physiotherapy Association (CPA) to 'respect the client's rights, dignity, needs, wishes and values' (CPA, 1989:3) certainly expresses worthy sentiments, but does not give specific guidance on how these sentiments should be reflected in specific situations. Perhaps in recognition of this difficulty, professional codes have increas-ingly been supplemented by more detailed guidance. The APTA *Code of Ethics* (APTA, 1991) is accompanied by a *Guide for Professional Conduct* (APTA, 1995), and the most recent *Rules of Professional Conduct* of the CSP, while occupying a single page in themselves, are contained within a booklet running to 48 pages (CSP, 1996b). The British Medical Association has long taken to publishing its ethical guidance in books rather than booklets (e.g. BMA, 1993).

There is, however, an underlying conflict between, on the one hand, providing a widely applicable guide to ethical conduct based on a putative professional consensus, and, on the other hand, providing advice on specific ethical problems. At one level, this is a reflection of the inability of general rules to legis-late for the detail and intricacy of concrete situations:

> No set of rules could encompass all the subtle complexities of even the most ordinary relationship between two persons, much less the special dimensions peculiar to the medical transaction in which one person in special need seeks the assistance of another who professes to help. (Pellegrino, 1979:51)

At another level, it can be suggested that a code of ethics represents an external, impersonal source of ethical guidance, whereas the ideals or principles of the individual practitioner are internal and personal. There are deep-rooted differences, and even incompatibilities, between the two:

> Neither aspect, taken alone, is really satisfactory as an ethic. The internal ethic is apt to be ill-formed, inarticulate, and crowded with subjective

and contradictory elements, more a personal expression of feelings than a set of examinable rules. As for the external aspect, it has been asked if a 'code of ethics' is not, all by itself, a contradiction in terms; as a set of rules that to outward appearances are to be applied more or less mechanically, it can hardly be adequate to the infinite variety of individual situations that present us with ethical dilemmas. Further, the two aspects, personal conscience and Code, work together with difficulty under the most stable conditions: it is of the essence of conscience to resist prior decision of cases by rules, which is precisely what a Code aims at doing. (Newton, 1981:45–6)

Benjamin and Curtis suggest that the generality of ethical codes allows practitioners who hold conflicting views to 'mask their differences by silently interpreting the code in accord with their favored position on various issues' (Benjamin and Curtis, 1986:7); however, when specific conflicts arise, these differences of opinion resurface, and the code is insufficient to settle the issue.

In the light of such considerations, Purtilo (1987a) suggests that a 'code of ethics' is perhaps better understood as a 'code of morality'. She takes 'morality' to refer, in a fairly non-specific way, to the moral principles to which a particular group or society attaches importance. 'Ethics', on the other hand, has more to do with the application of these principles, and encompasses such processes as:

to clarify the meaning of norms such as duties, to utilise methods of logic and other types of critical thinking systematically to think about how to resolve conflicts among the norms, and to give reasons for one's conclusions about how to proceed. (Purtilo, 1987a:33)

Hence, to describe a code as one of morality rather than ethics is to suggest that it functions to identify and highlight certain general moral values or principles, but does not necessarily provide specific aid to the therapist in critically analysing these values and principles and applying them systematically to concrete cases.

The problem may be more serious than this, however. A code of ethics may actually impede an analytical approach to ethics, for two reasons. First, the way in which it is made up of a series of fairly clear-cut rules, expressed in somewhat definitive terms, may encourage the practitioner to think that observing these rules is all that is required of him or her, and that there is no need for further reflection on the issues concerned. Accordingly, decisions on ethical questions may become mechanical and unreflective, and individual cases which are subtly but significantly different may be treated in a rather stereotyped manner. Further, categorical rules may cause therapists to overlook the fact that there are rarely any definitive answers in ethics: the morally right course of action in a particular situation is always an open question, and constant reappraisal of one's conduct is required.

Second, the focus of codes of ethics is almost exclusively on prescriptions and prohibitions, with little consideration given to matters of character traits. Accordingly, while ethical codes may provide a useful list of fairly general 'dos and don'ts', they do not really encourage the sort of moral virtue and ethical sensitivity seen to be important in Chapter 2. Feminist ethicists in particular are deeply distrustful of the role of codified morality, as they see it as excluding the emotional and interpersonal aspects of morality which are of particular importance in caring relationships (Noddings, 1984; Sherwin, 1992).

A certain amount can be done to offset the generality of codes of ethics by making them more detailed and providing explanatory notes to the various rules. However, a code that becomes very specific faces problems of its own:

> First, the code will not be able to avoid controversial precepts and hence will be unlikely to win widespread acceptance. Second, it will probably fill many thick volumes, and thus lose the advantages of brevity and simplicity. And third, no matter how detailed it is, such a code will always be incomplete if its aim is to give unambiguous guidance in all possible situations. (Benjamin and Curtis, 1986:7-8)

The fallibility of ethical codes

As has been stated, a code of ethics is the creation of the professional body. To a large extent, it serves as a public declaration of the collective moral standpoint of the profession, subject to revision from time to time. While the professional body is clearly well informed on the context and the technical nature of professional practice, it cannot claim any supreme authority on morality. As such, it is subject to conflict with the moral standpoints of other groups or individuals within society, and with morality in a general sense. Indeed, the ultimate test of a code of ethics is the extent to which it stands up to critical ethical scrutiny outside the confines of the profession.

It is misguided, therefore, to regard a code of ethics as the final arbiter of the moral correctness of professional conduct. Rather, it provides preliminary guidance which must be evaluated by the practitioner in the context of the situation at hand. As Johnstone points out, it is important

> to be especially vigilant not to fall prey to 'worshipping the code' at the expense of *being* ethical – and not to fall into the trap of treating the prescriptions and proscriptions of a code as absolute, and as ends in themselves, rather than as prima facie guides to ethical professional conduct. (Johnstone, 1994:46)

A code of ethics therefore has distinct limitations as an aid to moral reasoning and decision-making. This is not to say that one should expect ethical codes to be infallible – this would be an unreasonable and unrealistic demand – but it does highlight the fact that the code of ethics is not a substitute for critical and detailed ethical thinking by the individual practitioner. Moreover, such critical thinking should include an evaluation of the code of ethics itself.

The function of rules

Codes of ethics raise an important general issue about the role of rules within ethical decision-making. Moral rules are, of course, not restricted to codified morality. It was noted in Chapter 2 that fairly general prescriptions and prohibitions can be found in deontological frameworks, as secondary duties or principles. Equally, it was pointed out that consequentialism may advocate the following of certain general rules of conduct, based on the idea that this will have the best consequences in the long run, even if not on each specific occasion.

How useful, then, are moral rules in the sort of ethical decision-making therapists are likely to engage in? One of the criticisms that was made of ethical codes is that they are insensitive to the specific details and nuances of the individual case. It can be argued that, just as basic principles such as beneficence and non-maleficence need to be examined and weighed in specific circumstances, and not applied in a categorical and uncritical manner, so the injunctions of a code of ethics need to be analysed and evaluated on a case-by-case basis. However, a moment's reflection reveals that this is rather unrealistic. In Chapter 1 it was argued that a whole range of everyday activities in therapy practice have ethical implications. If therapists were to engage in a detailed ethical analysis of each of these, they would scarcely have time for anything else. In addition, in the busy world of health care, decisions on many courses of action have to be taken rapidly, with little time for conscious deliberation in the sort of detail that we are presently considering. It would seem, therefore, that there is an alternative recommendation to be made: instead of trying to analyse the specific details of each case from scratch, therapists might be better off following a set of general rules which will guide them in behaving ethically in their busy everyday practice. This is not to say that these rules should be followed in a totally unreflective, automatic manner, but simply that a detailed process of decision-making should not be attempted.

Which of these approaches should we adopt? Should we rely on a set of manageable rules, or should we judge each situation on its merits? Philosophers such as Richard Hare (1981) would argue that we should do both, because most of the time we are more likely to make the correct decision if we follow certain rules of conduct with which we are well acquainted, and which we can therefore internalize. If we were to work each case out in detail, this would not only be very time-consuming, but owing to our own deliberative shortcomings we might often reach a worse decision than if we were simply to 'follow the rules'. However, if we do nothing but observe a set of general rules, our ethical conduct is likely to become fossilized. From time to time, we need to reflect on our conduct, and subject it to detailed critical analysis. Similarly, some situations are simply too complex or unfamiliar to be dealt with by a set of rules. In these 'hard cases', we need to start at first principles and reach a conclusion that is specific to the details of the situation in question.

Accordingly, the therapist who says that 'ethical decision-making is fine, but there's simply not time for it' is misunderstanding exactly what is involved. Certainly, many decisions have to be taken on a more or less instinctive basis, in order to get

Table 8.1 Characteristics of case-specific and rule-based approaches to ethical decision-making

Case-by-case analysis	Following general rules
Time-consuming	Rapid
Complex and potentially exhausting	Relatively simple and effortless
Allows re-evaluation of ethical conduct	May lead to unreflective and stereotyped ethical conduct
Required for 'hard' cases	Probably sufficient for 'routine' cases

through the day's work, and not to be paralysed by indecision. However, there is a need, when time is available, to reappraise one's actions in these apparently routine situations. Moreover, when the therapist encounters those situations which raise particularly difficult problems – which occur infrequently, but perhaps more commonly than we think – following rules is insufficient and a much more detailed and thorough process of decision-making is needed.

Thus, an approach to ethics based on rules has much to recommend it, but it must be supplemented by a more analytical and reflective process. The key features of the two approaches we have been considering are summarized in Table 8.1.

Conclusion

Many of the comments in this chapter have been critical of codes of ethics. This is as it should be, and merely reflects the fact that the professions themselves are prepared to reconsider and revise their own codes. However, to be critical of certain features of ethical codes is not the same as dismissing them. On the contrary, such codes have an important part to play in the therapy professions, and this chapter will close with a brief statement of the role which codes of ethics can and should play in professional practice. In sum, the following would seem to be useful functions of the code of ethics:

- It alerts practitioners, in a general manner, to the need to take a moral perspective on therapy practice. The very existence of a code of ethics serves as a reminder that health care is a moral, not just a technical, enterprise.

- Having highlighted the importance of this moral perspective on practice, the code can indicate the general ethical values – such as respect for autonomy – which should characterize therapists' dealings with their clients.
- A code can provide a set of general prescriptions and prohibitions which may provide useful guidance for 'routine' decision-making.
- Although the ability of a code of ethics to deal with the detail of specific ethical issues may be limited, its promulgation may stimulate debate and critical reflection within the profession on such issues.
- A code of ethics may provide a useful medium through which to teach students about ethical issues (Banks, 1995), provided this is accompanied by an explanation of the nature and methods of ethical decision-making (Hussey, 1996).
- The code can signal specific practices that are deemed to be morally unacceptable, such as discrimination. Hence the APA document declares that physiotherapists are 'morally obliged to help all those who seek their professional services, regardless of age, gender, race, condition, nationality, creed, politics, financial and social status' (APA, 1990:118).
- A code can provide a clear statement of the basis on which disciplinary action may be taken by the professional body. This provides the practitioner with an indication of what professional repercussions may follow certain action (whether such action is morally justified or not).
- Codes of ethics provide a declaration to the public of professional values. Speaking of codes in nursing, Johnstone points out that they express 'the kinds of moral standards and values that patients and the broader community can expect nurses to uphold, and against which nurses can be held accountable' (Johnstone, 1994:47).
- Codes of ethics can potentially provide therapists with support in challenging managerial, institutional or statutory actions which are contrary to client welfare (Tschudin, 1992). However, this may require a greater emphasis within such codes on the wider social responsibilities of therapists, in addition to the predominant focus on aspects of the one-to-one therapeutic relationship.

9

Other topics: advocacy, suicide, care of older people, and HIV infection

In this chapter, a number of ethical issues will be examined in relation to specific situations or client groups. The general issues concerned will, for the most part, be ones that have already been examined in preceding chapters, but these will appear in especially sharp focus, or assume a particular importance, in the situations that follow. First, the question of advocacy will be examined. Following this, ethical issues relating to three client groups will briefly be addressed: clients at risk of suicide, the allocation of care to older people, and caring for HIV-positive clients.

Advocacy

Throughout this book, the concept of autonomy has been seen to be central to health care generally, and to therapy in particular. It has also been observed that the ability of patients and clients to exercise autonomy on their own behalf may be limited by a range of factors. Some of these factors are internal, such as age or cognitive and communication disorders, whereas others are external, such as the nature of the power relationships that exist between clients and professionals. A strategy that has developed to protect and promote the autonomy of clients in such situations is that of advocacy. Central to the idea of advocacy is an acknowledgment of the essential vulnerability of many patients and clients (Copp, 1986), and the disparity in power that exists between them and health care providers (Melia, 1989).

Within the law, advocacy has a specific meaning and is governed by particular legal procedures. For some professionals, such as social workers, the legal aspects of advocacy are of considerable importance. In therapy, however, advocacy is primarily an ethical concern. Advocacy can be broadly defined as:

> A process whereby one person undertakes to represent the wishes, decisions or interests of another person who is in some way restricted in, or prevented from, doing so on his or her own behalf.

Although advocacy is traditionally framed in terms of the client's autonomy, the above definition deliberately includes the possibility of acting as an advocate in the furtherance of other client interests, based perhaps on considerations of beneficence or justice. Within the role of advocate, there are two main activities open to the therapist:

> Advocacy is based on the notion of enabling users to articulate their needs and ensuring that their rights are respected. When users are unable to speak for themselves and do not have the capacity to decide what type of needs they have or how they would like them to be met, then the advocate will have to act in what is judged to be their best interests. (Banks, 1995:111)

The first of these, which may usefully be termed 'weak' advocacy, has to do with empowering clients and facilitating their expression of their own autonomy. This may involve helping clients to clarify their own values and wishes, making their rights known to them, and providing the information necessary to make certain choices. In the second form of activity, 'strong' advocacy, the advocate acts on behalf of the client, based upon an assessment of the client's best interests; instead of facilitating action by the client, the practitioner acts in the client's place.

A special case of advocacy is a practice known as 'whistle-blowing'. This is where a health care worker makes known the incompetent or unethical conduct of another practitioner or an institution, which threatens the welfare of patients or clients (Hunt, 1995). A form of 'strong' advocacy is often appropriate here, as clients themselves often have no means of knowing of the practices in question or, if they are aware of them, may be totally powerless to alter them.

MacLaren (1996) provides a discussion of advocacy which underlines its role in furthering the client's interests by some sort of intervention on the part of the professional. Less emphasis is given, however, to the fact that advocacy generally involves a third party; the therapist represents the client's wishes or interests to another professional, or makes the client's situation known to society in general.

The therapist as advocate

Most of the literature on advocacy in health care relates to the nursing profession, and Johnstone (1994) points out that some nurse theorists regard advocacy as in some sense the special prerogative of the nurse. However, the therapist is also well poised to assume this role, as the following examples illustrate (see also the case of Fleur Jacobs in Chapter 3):

> A speech and language therapist learns from a patient who has undergone a stroke that she has agreed to take part in a trial of hypertension therapy. Knowing that the patient's ability to communicate is markedly impaired following the stroke, the therapist doubts that the patient adequately understood what she was consenting to.

> An occupational therapist working on a psychiatric admissions ward is taking part in a case conference which is considering the possible discharge of a patient with depression. The patient himself is not present at the conference, and it seems that very little account is being taken of his own desires and preferences.

> A patient with multiple sclerosis is being rehabilitated at an out-patient facility. He is perceived by most of the rehabilitation team as being 'non-compliant', and the director of the unit has proposed that his programme of treatment should shortly be discontinued. The physiotherapist on the unit feels that the patient's unwillingness to engage fully in therapeutic activities is due to their perceived irrelevance to his normal lifestyle and activities.

> A physiotherapist working on a medical admissions ward is increasingly convinced that one of her colleagues is providing inadequate treatment

to patients admitted with acute respiratory impairment. Her colleague's treatments seem to be brief, cursory, and are often given at irregular and infrequent intervals. When challenged tactfully about this on more than one occasion, the other therapist responds aggressively and refuses to discuss the matter.

The limitations of advocacy

The idea of the therapist acting as an advocate for his or her patients is, on the face of it, an extremely attractive one. However, Johnstone (1994:273) points out that the 'validity and moral force of advocacy has [sic] been, in a somewhat question-begging fashion, merely assumed rather than critically determined', and argues for a more searching analysis of some of the conceptual and ethical difficulties to which the notion of advocacy may give rise. This section will examine some of the criticisms that can be levelled at the role of client advocate and the overall concept of advocacy.

The question of a mandate

Although the advocate seeks to act in the best interests of the client, in many cases he or she has not been chosen by the client for this role (Allmark and Klarzynski, 1992). Indeed, the very fact that the client is not competent to make such choices may be the reason that advocacy is seen to be appropriate. It follows that, unless they have been specifically requested by the client to fulfil this function, therapists must not assume that they have any unique authority to plead the client's case.

The danger of paternalism

The 'strong' form of advocacy defined earlier can clearly lead to paternalistic intervention on the part of therapists if they underestimate the client's ability to voice his or her own wishes, or pursue their own view of the client's interests instead of that which could reasonably be inferred to be the client's own. The questions of competence and substituted judgement discussed in Chapter 4 are crucial here.

Problems of 'dissociation'

In order to represent the client's interests fully and faithfully, therapists may have to discard their own professional perceptions, values, allegiances and vested interests. There is surely a limit to how far this is possible. Although therapists may endeavour to empathize with the client as much as possible, the strong processes of socialization through which they have passed is likely to have imbued them with certain strongly held values and assumptions. This may ensure that the 'professional' perspective will ultimately prevail over the 'lay'.

Problems of divided loyalties

The role of the therapist is often characterized by split loyalties (Bruckner, 1987), and advocacy exemplifies this problem clearly. In addition to their responsibilities to their clients, therapists have loyalties to colleagues, to the institution in which they work, and to their profession as a whole. These professional allegiances may conflict with their loyalties to the client: indeed, the need for advocacy may arise specifically because there is an incompatibility between client and professional interests.

Ultimately, the question arises: 'at what point in a caring relationship does the professional role of the nurse compromise the advocate role, or alternatively the role of advocate compromise the professional role?' (Gates, 1994:16). It is perhaps reasonable to think that, in many cases, professional loyalties will ultimately tend to be favoured by the therapist, if only subconsciously. Making a stand for the client against colleagues or the health care institution may have undesirable personal or professional repercussions for the therapist, and there will thus be a strong prudential reason to avoid this if possible. At the very least, a whole-hearted pursuit of advocacy will always be constrained by these potentially incompatible professional priorities.

This line of argument gives rise to a further difficulty. If therapist advocates are to represent the interests of the client against potentially paternalistic, intrusive or harmful actions on the part of other health professionals, how are they to be sure that what they take to be advocacy for the client is not just a subconscious form of precisely the same professional interference? Therapists may find it very hard to gain a view of the client's interests which is not influenced by their own professional values and assumptions – in which case, presumably, the client's interests are unlikely to be authentically represented, and the need for advocacy remains.

Advocacy as potentially self-serving

Advocacy frequently brings the advocate into some degree of opposition or conflict with other professionals, and the practitioner may seek a greater degree of professional power in order more effectively to fulfil the role of advocate. Bernal (1992) questions the legitimacy of this combining of professional aspirations with an avowed protection of patients' rights. In such a process, heightened professional autonomy is sought as a means of furthering client autonomy. It is not clear that the two forms of autonomy are wholly compatible – can therapists empower themselves at the same time as seeking to empower clients? Indeed, there is a danger that the process of advocacy will become one of professional rivalry. The client may therefore be overlooked as therapists seek to establish their legitimacy or authority in the eyes of other professionals – or worse still, the client may become a pawn in this process (Allmark and Klarzynski, 1992; Bird, 1994; Johnstone, 1994).

The questionable distinctness of advocacy within ethics

Johnstone (1994) points out that advocacy is often proposed as a distinct moral activity within health care, qualitatively different from other aspects of health care ethics. She queries whether this is the case. It may be that advocacy is merely a particular means of honouring such moral principles as respect for autonomy, beneficence, and so forth. This would certainly seem to be the case in respect of 'weak' advocacy. In other words, advocacy is not necessarily a special area of moral activity which therapists may or may not decide to engage in – it is, perhaps, merely an extension of their usual moral duties to situations in which there may be reluctance on the part of others to respect the client's interests or welfare.

Conclusion

Despite the misgivings expressed in the previous section, there would seem to be a legitimate place for the sorts of action that are encompassed by advocacy, whether or not they are seen as distinct from other ethical responsibilities of the therapist. There are, however, three caveats:

- 'Strong' advocacy should be reserved for cases in which clients' ability to voice their own wishes is clearly impaired, or areas which lie outside clients' sphere of knowledge (such as cases of whistleblowing); otherwise, the therapist's intervention risks being paternalistic.
- The temptation to use advocacy as a means of professional advancement, either individual or collective, should be firmly resisted.
- Consideration should be given, where appropriate, to the use of independent advocates, who do not have prior allegiances to either professional or client.

The client at risk of suicide

Suicide is a relatively common occurrence. Beauchamp and Childress (1994) estimate that there are 30 000 certified suicides each year in the USA. Many other probable suicides are not classed as such, either because the exact circumstances of the death are insufficiently clear-cut to justify a formal declaration of suicide, or in order to protect the feelings and legal interests of surviving family members.

Definitions

How is suicide to be defined? Brown *et al.* offer the following definition: 'Suicide occurs when an individual determines to kill himself or herself and succeeds in doing so' (Brown *et al.*, 1992:161). A somewhat fuller definition is provided by Fairbairn:

> Suicide is an act, whether of commission or omission, and whether performed by himself or others, by means of which an individual autonomously intends and wishes to bring about his death because he wants to be dead or wants to die the death he enacts. (Fairbairn, 1995:84)

In addition, there is what is known as 'attempted suicide'. This covers several varieties of apparently intended non-fatal self-harm:

> [I]t is used in referring to suicides that have failed, occasions when a person has intentionally self harmed in a way that could have led to death but was unsure whether he wished to die, occasions where an individual has aimed to create the illusion that he intended to die though he actually intended to live, and occasions where a person's brush with death was accidental. (Fairbairn, 1995:40–1)

Glover suggests that some attempts at suicide represent a firm decision to die, some are a cry for help with no firm intention to die, while others may represent 'a state of mind where a gamble is taken with some risk of death and some chance of survival followed by help' (Glover, 1977:172). Clearly, there are a number of situations which fall under the general heading of suicidal action.

Suicide has been decriminalized in most states of the USA (Brock, 1993), and since the Suicide Act 1961, committing suicide is no longer a criminal offence in the UK (Mason and McCall Smith, 1994). Assisting suicide, however, remains illegal.

Moral conflicts for the therapist

For most therapists, suicide, or attempted suicide, is not a routine occurrence within their everyday clinical practice. However, those working in psychiatry – especially in acute care settings – are likely to encounter clients who have tried, or will try, to end their own lives. Less frequently, the situation will arise in a non-psychiatric setting:

> Jack Harvey is a 35-year-old man who sustained an incomplete mid-cervical spinal injury 18 months ago in a motorcycle accident. He now relies upon an electric wheelchair. With the use of a number of assistive

devices, he can perform some minor activities of self-care, but is largely dependent upon his wife and his sister, with whom he lives. Prior to the accident, he had been a very successful fashion photographer, but is now totally unable to pursue his career. Anna Kaminski is an occupational therapist at the spinal injuries unit to which Jack was first admitted, and has been involved with his management ever since. Jack returns to the unit regularly for functional assessments, and Anna has got to know him very well. It has become clear to her that Jack has not adapted to his disability; indeed, he often seems to be extremely pessimistic about his future life. During one visit to the unit, Jack seems particularly depressed, and lets it slip to Anna that he often thinks of suicide. He even indicates that he has worked out 'the best way to do it'. At this point, he changes the subject, and begs Anna not to tell anyone about their conversation: 'I don't want you telling anybody else in the unit about this, and I certainly don't want Joanne or Rosemary [his wife and his sister] to hear about it'. Anna tries to persuade Jack to talk to her more about the subject, but he refuses.

In a situation such as this, a number of options are open to Anna Kaminski. First, she can let the matter drop and forget about it; however, she feels that this is simply to 'duck the issue', and does not regard it as a serious option. She then considers telling the consultant, so that a psychiatric consultation can be arranged. Anna reasons that it is her duty to obtain help for Jack, but she does not feel she is qualified to provide such help herself. She realizes, however, that enlisting help would mean breaking a confidence. Anna also thinks of telling Jack's wife, who would be able to take steps to prevent Jack from killing himself, or at least minimize the chances of his doing so. This too, however, would involve a breach of confidentiality. Hence, Anna finds herself in an apparent dilemma. On the one hand, to repeat the details of her conversation to anyone else would be to go against Jack's wishes. On the other hand, to remain silent would be to fail in her perceived duty to help Jack.

A solution to this impasse requires a number of fundamental questions to be answered. First, is Jack's apparent intention to commit suicide a genuine one? Some consider that many people who declare their intention to kill themselves, or attempt unsuccessfully to do so, are in fact making a 'cry for help'. Fairbairn (1995) suggests that while some threats of suicide may indicate a determination to commit suicide, the intention is often to induce a response on the part of others. If Jack is actually seeking help, then perhaps he is not really asking for confidentiality, but is implicitly asking Anna to alert others to his situation. How is Anna to know whether Jack's intention is real? It may be that a psychiatric opinion is required to settle the issue. However, this would involve breaking a confidence, whereas the whole purpose of assessing the authenticity of Jack's intention is to determine whether breaching confidentiality is permissible in the first place.

Assuming that Jack's wish to die is authentic, a separate question arises: is this an autonomous, rational intention? It may be felt that a desire for suicide is by definition an irrational desire – and probably evidence of some sort of psychopathology (Ringel, 1980). On this view, nobody who can reason rationally would choose to die. In a similar way, some writers on health care ethics seem to assume that suicide is necessarily an action that 'harms' the individual, and therefore justifies action to prevent it:

> The avoidance of certain harm befalling the person about to be deceived would outweigh the general principle of truthfulness that should operate in professional relationships. There would be no difficulty in defending the decision to tell the person poised to commit suicide a lie that can be expected to stop the person from committing an irrevocable act of self-destruction. (Schröck, 1980:145)

Of course, the person committing suicide is indeed harmed, in the literal sense of this word. However, if we carry the principle of *volenti non fit injuria* ('no injury is done to someone who consents') across from the law, it can be argued that people who truly wish to die are not really harming themselves, as the action is in accordance with their own interests (even though it admittedly puts an end to the pursuit of any future interests).

In contrast to this sort of standpoint, there is a growing appreciation that there is such thing as 'rational suicide' (Heyd and Bloch, 1991). Accordingly, we have to ask, first of all, whether or not it is possible for a person to make a rational choice for suicide, and therefore act autonomously in ending his or her life. If we feel that this is indeed possible, we must then ask whether the case in hand is an example of such autonomous action.

If it is thought that Jack is behaving autonomously in expressing a wish to die, then to interfere might be seen as paternalistic; his own autonomous wishes are overridden for the sake of somebody else's conception of his good. It must be remembered that just because we do not regard somebody's actions as *reasonable*, this is not to say that they are necessarily *irrational*. The standard for rationality is much the same for everybody, but that of reasonableness is related to the particular values and priorities of the individual. If, however, Anna does *not* interfere, then Jack is permitted to pursue his own chosen course of action, with due respect for his autonomy.

In contrast, if Jack is not behaving autonomously, then a decision to forestall a suicide attempt will not, by definition, interfere with his self-determination, whereas taking no action may allow him to die without having made an autonomous choice to do so – Anna will have failed to protect his welfare, and may understandably feel that she has failed in her moral duty. The various alternatives here are summarized in Figure 9.1.

In relation to both the question of distinguishing a genuine wish to die from a cry for help and that of judging the autonomy of an attempted suicide, the problem arises as to how to assess these questions correctly. As we have seen, invoking psychiatric help may effectively pre-empt the issue. Given that there is frequently some doubt on such questions, even with expert advice, one solution is to consider the various possible consequences of the available courses of action, and steer clear of the

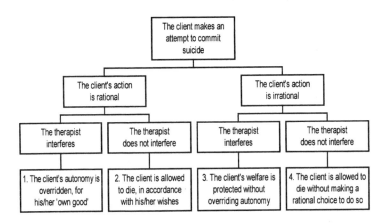

Figure 9.1 Alternative responses to a client who attempts suicide, depending on the rationality of the decision

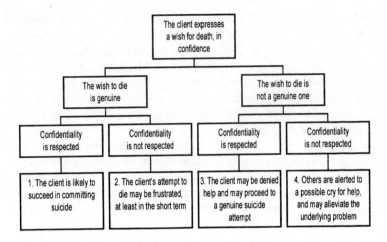

Figure 9.2 Alternative responses to a client who expresses a wish to die, depending on the genuineness of the wish to die

worst possible outcome: a 'safer bet' strategy is adopted. If we examine Figure 9.1, the worst outcome would seem to be that the client is permitted to die without having consciously made this choice (outcome 4 in Figure 9.1). Thus, if there is a suggestion that the client is acting irrationally, it is safer to interfere than not to. Similarly, if we return to the question of a genuine wish to die and examine Figure 9.2, the worst outcome would seem to be respecting confidentiality when the wish to die is not genuine (outcome 3 in Figure 9.2). Accordingly, if a cry for help is suspected, the safest course of action will normally be to take action to provide help to the client; as this is likely to involve enlisting the help of other professionals, it will usually involve breaching confidentiality. However, given the grave potential consequences of not providing professional help in such a situation, the breaking of a confidence may be felt to be justified, in terms of the discussion of this issue in Chapter 5.

However, if Anna is confident that the client's wish to die is genuine, and has good reason for thinking this, she might feel impelled to maintain confidentiality, for in this way she would respect Jack's autonomy in terms of both his wish to die and his desire for confidentiality (outcome 1 in Figure 9.2). Similarly, to revert to the question of rationality and autonomy, if Anna is convinced, on reasonable grounds, that Jack is rational, she may justifiably decide not to interfere in the furtherance of his suicidal intentions (outcome 2 in Figure 9.1). However, in both cases, given the irrevocable nature of the suicidal act, the onus would be on Anna to take all reasonable steps, short of breaching confidentiality, to establish that Jack is indeed rational, and that he really does intend to die rather than simply to seek help.

It should also be remembered that not all 'interference' is contrary to respecting the client's autonomy. Fairbairn (1995) suggests that there are three stages of intervention: discussion of the person's intentions and wishes, persuasion, and coercive intervention. It could be argued that, far from being paternalistic, discussion with the would-be suicide is a means of promoting the individual's autonomy, by encouraging him or her to examine the nature and motivation of the proposed action. Similarly, as was noted in Chapter 4, persuasion only conflicts with respect for autonomy when it reaches a certain stage and crosses over into a form of verbal duress. In the case of coercive intervention, however, autonomy is liable to be overridden. Removing all means of death from the autonomous individual would fall under this heading, as would physically preventing an attempt at suicide – and a breach of confidentiality which led to either of these would be equivalent.

Certain other issues are raised by this case, which it is worth discussing briefly. Hitherto, the implicit focus has been on whether Jack's wish to die should be disclosed to other members of staff in the unit. However, there is also the question as to whether Anna should say anything to Jack's wife or his sister. It is almost certain that they would wish to be warned, and would possibly seek to prevent Jack from carrying out his intention – given Jack's functional limitations, they would most likely succeed in doing so. Additionally, in the event of Jack's committing suicide, they are likely to experience great distress, and perhaps feelings of guilt also.

However, health professionals have to consider carefully to whom their primary duties are owed. It is reasonable to argue that their priority is to further the interests of the client, and that while the interests of relatives should also be promoted as far as possible, these must take second place. After all, if we follow the argument proposed in Chapter 6 that a person's life cannot be ended purely in order to satisfy the wishes of others, it seems equally clear that we cannot use the wishes of others forcibly to prolong the life of somebody who no longer desires to live. Thus, if it is concluded that Jack has the autonomy-based right to take his own life, and that warning his family of this possibility is likely to frustrate any attempt he may make on his own life, there may be a moral requirement to say nothing.

If, on the other hand, Jack is thought to be expressing a non-autonomous wish, then warning his family is likely to be a means not of frustrating but of protecting his interests, and to this extent will be morally appropriate.

The case we have been considering is one in which advance warning is given of the individual's suicidal intentions. In some instances, no such warning is given. For example, a community therapist might call on a patient and discover that he or she has taken an overdose of sleeping tablets; although there is no sign of a suicide note, it appears to be a case of attempted suicide. In such a case, immediate intervention to save the patient's life is appropriate in order to provide the opportunity of investigating the circumstances of the case and examining the patient's state of mind. Until such time as the patient's autonomy can be unambiguously confirmed, considerations of beneficence demand that help is sought.

Finally, the emotional and psychological impact of suicide on the therapist must be acknowledged. A variety of responses may occur:

- The therapist may feel intense concern for the individual, and undergo considerable personal distress and anguish on his or her behalf.
- The practitioner may feel a strong desire to help, but may find that help is not wanted or, whether desired or not, is ineffective in changing the client's resolve, with resulting feelings of inadequacy, failure and guilt.
- The therapist may have firm religious or personal moral objections to the idea of self-killing and find it hard to empathize with the would-be suicide – a strong sense of moral disapproval may (though it need not necessarily) displace sympathy and understanding.

Conclusion

The issue of suicide illustrates vividly the ethical difficulties that may arise in connection with the issues of competence and paternalism. Dealing with a suicidal client may be an emotionally stressful experience, and therapists should do all that they can to support one another in such situations. It should be remembered, however, that the choice that causes the therapist the least anguish is not thereby the morally correct course of action – the 'easy' option for the professional may be the 'hard' option for the client.

The allocation of care to older patients

It has been commented that 'the medical care of individuals in old age bristles with issues which require consideration from an ethical point of view' (Jeffreys, 1993). Perhaps the most pressing of these concerns resource allocation, and many of the issues previously touched upon in Chapter 7 in relation to this topic are vividly highlighted in the case of elderly people. In view of the large proportion of their time that therapists spend caring for this section of the population, it is worth examining some of the specific issues that arise.

Issues of resource allocation have become crystallized with respect to elderly people because of two related facts:

1   The growing proportion of the population in industrialized societies that is elderly.
2   The increasing demands that these members of society are making on health care resources. (Jette and Bottomley, 1987; Guccione, 1988b)

Recent changes in the demographic profile in Western societies have been dramatic. In the UK, the proportion of the population over 65 is likely to increase from a present figure of 18 per cent to a figure of 30 per cent by the year 2030 (Rivlin, 1995). Correspondingly, Callahan (1991) points out that, according to some projections, by the year 2040 the elderly will represent 21 per cent of the USA population and will account for 45 per cent of all health care expenditure. There are clearly important financial reasons to consider the allocation of health care resources to elderly people. Equally, there are important ethical reasons to ensure that the distribution of resources to or from these citizens, at either the 'macro' or the 'micro' level, is just.

Age as the basis for resource allocation

It is sometimes suggested that age should be used as a criterion for withholding, limiting, or rationing health care. The cost of providing care for an increasing elderly population has prompted some to argue for curtailment of treatment for this portion of the population. Richard Lamm, a former governor of the state of Colorado, argues:

> It is not only fair but desirable to have a different level of care for a 10-year-old than for someone who is 100. Should not public policy recognize that some people have far more statistical years ahead of them than others? I feel it is morally repugnant to use $100,000 or more of our kids' limited resources, as I'm on my way out the door. (cited in Waymack, 1991:249)

However, as with any arguments directed at limiting care for certain categories of people, it is important to guard against unjustifiable forms of discrimination. Where older people are concerned, the need to do so is especially acute in view of the prevalence of ageist attitudes in Western society. Ageism can be regarded as a set of attitudes, beliefs and practices directed at certain members of society on the basis of their chronological age. Crucially, the beliefs concerned are generally stereotypical (i.e. overgeneralized and exaggerated, with little appreciation of the variation in attributes and abilities which may be present within a particular category); the attitudes in question are usually negative (i.e. embodying various forms of social, moral or aesthetic denigration); and the resulting practices are generally discriminatory (i.e. involving various forms of unjustifiably disadvantageous treatment). While ageism can in theory be applied to those on any part of the age spectrum, it is almost invariably directed at older people. Bytheway and Johnson argue that, in terms of its impact on society, ageism 'legitimates' the use of chronological age to mark out classes of people who are systematically denied resources and opportunities that others enjoy, and who suffer the consequences of such denigration – ranging from well-meaning patronage to unambiguous vilification. (Bytheway and Johnson, 1990:37)

Bell further argues that any discrimination against older people in the allocation of health care resources is also a form of indirect discrimination against women, given that 'there are many more elderly women than there are elderly men, and these older women are poorer, more apt to live long, and less likely to have informal social and personal supports than their male counterparts' (Bell, 1992:85).

With these ideas in mind, we can examine three arguments which may be advanced to justify age-based resource allocation in health care.

Let nature take its course

The view is sometimes expressed that whereas illness and disability in younger people are biological aberrations which should be corrected, loss of health in later life is a normal part of the ageing process: illness in youth is unnatural and avoidable, in old age it is natural and inevitable. Consequently, it may be felt that there is a correspondingly greater moral imperative to provide health care for younger people. Indeed, excessive medical intervention in the lives of older people may be seen as interfering with nature in a morally reprehensible manner.

There are several difficulties with this sort of view. In the first place, determining what is 'natural' is a far from straightforward business. With the scientific and technological advances that have been made, particularly in this current century, it is hard to know exactly what the natural course of events would look like. In any case, many philosophers would argue that examining what occurs in the external world does not produce the answer to moral questions. This is to confuse 'what is' with 'what should be'; not everything which occurs naturally is necessarily a good thing.

Even if the idea of allowing events to proceed naturally is accepted, it would seem arbitrary to classify ill-health in younger life as 'unnatural' and that in old age as 'natural', and then take the decision on whether or not to provide care and treatment on this basis. A case could probably be made that some illnesses experienced by young adults are more 'natural' than some of those experienced by older people, with the result that the young adults would be the ones to forgo treatment. A far more coherent and consistent position would be to regard virtually all ill-health as natural, and leave it all untreated!

This appeal to nature also tends to misconstrue the consequences of letting disease and illness take their own course in elderly people. Advances in medicine, nutrition and sanitation have meant that the last years of life may consist of prolonged discomfort and incapacity:

> Hence, any notion that denial of treatment to the elderly will simply allow a return to the more 'natural' modes of death enjoyed by earlier, simpler generations is a dangerously romanticized misconception. To ration health care by denial of treatment is not simply to abandon the patient to death but, often, to abandon him to a prolonged period of morbidity, only later followed by death. (Battin, 1994:66)

Thus, we should be aware of exactly what effects a denial of treatment to older people may have on their lives.

The idea of 'letting nature take its course' is fraught with difficulties, and does not provide a sound basis for the allocation of care.

There is little 'return' on treatment

This argument is based on the advantage that accrues from treating older people, and may take two forms:

1   Older people themselves do not benefit greatly from therapeutic input.
2   Regardless of whether individual older people benefit from treatment, there is negligible overall resulting benefit for society.

According to Rivlin (1995), the first proposition is at least partially false. He cites work by Brandstetter (1992) and Jecker and Schneiderman (1992) which shows that age is often a poor predictor of, and may even be irrelevant to, an individual's response to many forms of treatment, including major interventions such as coronary bypass surgery and liver and kidney transplantation. On a more general note, Hunt points out that to use age alone as a medical indicator is misguided:

> Chronology indicates virtually nought about other more important clinical considerations, such as the patient's quality of life, the amenability of a condition to treatment and the expressed wishes of the patient and family. It would be unrealistic and simplistic to ascribe age absolute preeminence in all life-death clinical decision-making relating to elderly persons. (Hunt, 1993:22)

In addition, quite apart from its factual or predictive basis, a criterion based on 'ability to benefit' could be used to restrict treatment to all sorts of patients, young as well as old, in whom there is limited scope for clinical improvement. The young child with incurable cancer of the pineal gland would be as vulnerable to such reasoning as the septuagenarian with end-stage cardiac failure.

The second proposition to be examined – that society does not benefit from the treatment of older people – is also problematic. Shaw suggests that there is an economic argument for directing care to younger members of society, in that it is 'in the interest of the old people of the future to spend more keeping the young and the working healthy than the retired' (Shaw, 1994:188). The logic of this is questionable. If resources are to be directed preferentially to the young, this suggests that these younger members of society will only benefit *now*; when they themselves become the old people of the future, they will be the victims, not the beneficiaries, of such a policy. Nonetheless, it is true that, in one sense, older people are no longer fully productive members of society; they are mostly retired and probably make little direct financial contribution to the community. However, productivity can take other forms. Older people play a valuable role in the social and emotional life of the family, and French (1997) points out that they play a significant part in informal care. Older people may also be very active in the cultural and intellectual life of society; here, French (1997) and Rivlin (1995) cite examples such as Pablo Picasso and Bertrand Russell. Whatever their present input, it should be remembered that most old people have a lifetime of financial contribution to society – through taxes, and such like – behind them. It seems rather arbitrary that we should only consider future contributions when seeking to balance this particular account. Indeed, these past contributions are already securely in place, whereas the future contributions of the young are only potential (Battin, 1994). Moreover, some young people, such as severely physically disabled children, have very little prospect of making any future financial contribution to society, and may be a net recipient of societal resources for decades to come. The present argument would serve to exclude them from treatment even more effectively than it would many older people.

The 'fair innings' argument

This argument proposes that priority should be given to those who have only lived a small proportion of their natural lives; older people have already had a good allocation of life, and therefore have less claim on care, especially of a life-saving nature. Harris sums up the core of the 'fair innings' argument as follows:

> Let's say that a fair share of life is the traditional three score and ten, seventy years. Anyone who does not reach seventy suffers, on this view, the injustice of being cut off in their prime. They have missed out on a reasonable share of life; they have been short-changed. Those, however, who do make seventy suffer no such injustice, they have not lost out but rather must consider any additional years a sort of bonus beyond that which could reasonably be hoped for. The fair innings argument requires that everyone be given an equal chance to have a fair innings, to reach the appropriate threshold but, having reached it, they have received their entitlement. (Harris, 1985:91)

The underlying conception of justice here would seem to be that of 'to each an equal share'. It was suggested in Chapter 7 that this idea may not work if the different needs of individuals are such that an equal share is of unequal value to them. However, everybody presumably has an equal 'need' for life, so initially there does not seem to be anything in principle wrong with this approach to justice.

Perhaps the greatest problem with the fair innings argument is not so much with its philosophical basis as with its application. Once we have decided that a certain age threshold will determine the allocation of resources, according to Harris (1985) there is little justification for setting this threshold at 70 as opposed to, say, 40 or 50. Any particular threshold will tend to be a largely arbitrary choice. Even if we discard the notion of a specific threshold, and look at the difference in the amount of well-being that older patients have already enjoyed compared to younger patients (Veatch, 1988), it remains to be established at what point a difference in age becomes relevant. If we are to divert limited neurological rehabilitation facilities to a patient of 40 in preference to one of 75, should we not also give priority to a patient of 30 over one of 40? Even if the first act of prioritization seems reasonable, the second seems unacceptable. In other words, once we have accepted age as the deciding factor, it is hard to resist the conclusion that virtually *any* age difference should be a relevant consideration.

Another difficulty with this sort of view is that it seeks to impose an external value on other people's lives. In particular, it presumes that a longer expected lifespan is automatically more valuable than a shorter one. Lewis and Bottomley (1994) argue that it is the value of a life to the person whose life it is that is paramount. As we have previously noted when considering the QALY, trying to reach a comparative valuation of the lives of others is an invidious process, and is especially dangerous in respect of older people, given that they 'often have a different set of values in their assessments of the quality of life than do younger persons' (Macklin, 1982:122).

In relation to this and the preceding arguments, it can be seen that the use of age as a criterion of resource allocation is fraught with problems. This is not to say that age has *no* part to play in decisions on how to allocate care. Certainly in respect of efficiency, if not equity, life-expectancy may be a relevant consideration. However, if age is the dominant, or the sole, criterion of allocation, the amount of care which individuals receive (or even whether they receive care at all) will come to depend on a biological factor whose moral relevance is at best tenuous.

Conclusion

The fairest way to determine the allocation of resources to older patients is probably on the straightforward basis of need. There are, however, two important provisos here:

1   The calculation of need should be carried out with greater
    emphasis on immediate than on long-term predictions.
    Suppose that, in relation to their respective potential capaci-
    ties, one client of 75 and another of 48 both appear to be
    similarly functionally impaired. They should each be seen as
    having a more or less equal claim to rehabilitation, even
    though any functional improvement gained for the second
    client may be enjoyed for a greater number of years. The
    primary concern is with engineering a favourable change in
    the person's health status; the long-term duration of such a
    change, while not wholly ignored, is given less weight. In
    this way, one can at least partially avoid discriminating
    against older people on the basis of their age.

2   A problem which is common to both of the arguments
    which have just been reviewed is that they seem to discrimi-
    nate against older people, *as a group*, purely on the basis of
    their age, and thereby ignore the individuality of each client
    or patient. Where macroallocation has to be performed
    between different specialties, it is necessary to some degree
    to consider client groups. However, where decisions of
    microallocation are being made in respect of *individual*
    clients, the focus should be on the relevant needs of each
    person, rather than on the individual's membership of a
    crude category such as 'young' or 'old'. This will help to
    ensure that any denial of treatment to older people is in
    terms of factors which are relevant within the specific case
    in question, rather than in terms of a stereotypical view of
    what it is to be old.

A final point that is worth considering is that older people have
comparatively little power and influence in society. Although
elderly people can cast their votes in elections, and make their
voices heard in other ways, the fact remains that most positions of
influence and authority in society are occupied by young or
middle-aged adults. Equally, care of older people (especially long-
term care) has not hitherto enjoyed a high profile within health
care (Fortinsky, 1993). Hence, when it comes to determining the
allocation of health care resources, therapists may have a special
responsibility to press the interests of those who represent a
disempowered section of the community:

The requirement for health professionals to engage at the level of health policy will be unpalatable to many who do not like to get into the 'dirty work' of politics and government. Nonetheless, no greater challenge faces the health professional in the treatment of the elderly than that of becoming a voice for the all-too-often voiceless, assuring a fair allocation of health resources. (Purtilo, 1987b:180)

Caring for HIV-positive clients

Whereas many topics in health care ethics have been the subject of debate for many years, the recent AIDS pandemic has raised a variety of ethical issues which had hitherto received comparatively little scrutiny in the health care ethics literature. Physiotherapists, occupational therapists and speech and language therapists all have a role to play in the management of patients with AIDS (AOTA, 1989; Bakland *et al.*, 1989; Coates, 1990a; Atchison *et al.*, 1990; Cusack and Singh, 1994), and must therefore give careful consideration to the ethical context of their practice with this client group.

The current picture

There is no doubting the impact of HIV and AIDS. At the time of writing, up-to-date epidemiological data are being presented at an international conference on AIDS taking place in Vancouver. It is estimated that throughout the world 27 900 000 people have become HIV-infected since the first appearance of the virus, this total increasing by 8500 each day (Nau, 1996). In this

Table 9.1 Geographical distribution of cases of AIDS

Region	Cases of AIDS (%)
Africa	77
Europe	3
United States of America	7
America (excluding USA)	6
Asia	7
Oceania	<1

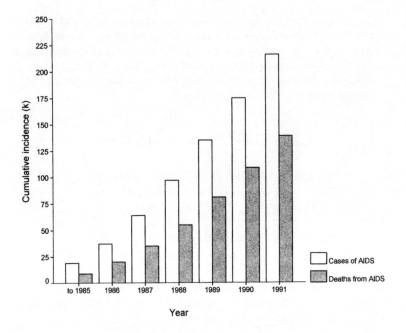

Figure 9.3 The cumulative incidence of cases of AIDS, and resultant deaths, in the USA up to 1991

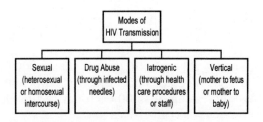

Figure 9.4 Modes of transmission of HIV

period, the number of cases of AIDS is thought to have reached nearly 8 000 000 worldwide, and their geographical distribution is shown in Table 9.1.

Since its arrival, the spread of AIDS has been dramatic. Figure 9.3 shows the cumulative incidence of cases of AIDS, and resultant deaths, in the USA up to 1991.

There are a number of ways in which HIV can be transmitted (Figure 9.4). These have in common the exchange, transmission or absorption of certain bodily fluids. The massive preponderance of cases of AIDS in Africa reflects the fact that, worldwide, sexual activity of a heterosexual nature is by far the principal mode of transmission (Pratt, 1995).

Ethical issues raised

These epidemiological facts are daunting, and their implications for health care and other aspects of public policy are considerable. However, the immediate ethical issues facing therapists are more practical ones. The principal ethical questions are:

- What do therapists need to know about their clients' HIV status?
- Should a client's HIV status be revealed to third parties?
- What do clients need to know about their therapists' HIV status?
- What bearing should clients' HIV status have on their care and treatment by therapists?

The last of these questions has been considered in detail elsewhere (Hansen, 1990; Sim and Purtilo, 1991; Sim, 1992) and will not be addressed here. The focus of this section will therefore be on the first three questions, though these will be examined fairly briefly, as many of the basic issues have already been explored in earlier chapters.

Who needs to know the client's HIV status?

The issue here is clearly one of confidentiality. The starting assumption is that information as to the health status of either clients or health professionals should remain privileged unless there are reasons of greater weight supporting its disclosure. Do such reasons exist in the case of HIV infection? There is evidence that therapists feel that they should know the HIV status of their clients (Dike, 1993; Falk-Kessler *et al.*, 1994), but does this rest on a sound basis? There are two possible reasons why therapists might feel that they should be aware of the HIV status of their clients:

1   Because it might determine the effectiveness of therapeutic interventions
2   Because the therapist, and others, might be at risk of infection.

The first of these reasons does not rest on a sound basis. It is certainly the case that therapists need to know what condition they are being asked to treat. However, uncomplicated HIV infection is not in itself treatable by therapists, and so there is no need to know on this count (admittedly, counselling is frequently given to those who are infected by the virus, but this is rarely the primary responsibility of the therapist). Individuals infected with HIV may, of course, be treated for other problems, but it is not clear, in most cases, that their being HIV-positive or not will determine the effectiveness of this treatment.

If the client has progressed to having AIDS, the situation is somewhat different. A number of features of this syndrome, both physical and psychological, are amenable to treatment or management by therapists – e.g. respiratory infections, neuro-muscular impairments, disturbances of mood, cognition and affect, and general fatigue and malaise. There may also be symptomatic conditions related to HIV infection which fall short of a formal diagnosis of AIDS. However, in such cases the diagnosis is almost certainly already known to the health care staff involved with the client's care, and the question of whether the therapist should know has already been settled.

Thus, in those cases (i.e. AIDS and certain sequelae of HIV infection) where therapists need to know the diagnosis for the purposes of effective intervention, the likelihood is that they already have this information, and in those cases where they may well not know the diagnosis (i.e. most cases of HIV infection prior to the development of AIDS), it can be argued that they do not need to know it.

The other argument – that therapists need to know for their own protection – is less straightforward. There are, however, a number of objections that can be raised against it. Above all, it is important to consider the nature of the therapeutic interaction likely to occur between therapist and client before deciding to what extent therapists need to be acquainted with their clients' HIV status. A comparison between therapists and other health professionals is instructive here. A surgeon working in the emergency room of a busy city-centre hospital, dealing with a large number of gunshot wounds and road accident injuries, is likely to come into frequent contact with patients' blood (Gerberding *et al.*, 1990). Possible skin puncture while suturing or using a scalpel may lead to inoculation with infected plasma. Although there are some areas of therapy practice where contact with blood or open wounds may occur – such as treatment of burns, wound debridement, postoperative care, percutaneous electromyography (Latourette, 1992) – the likelihood of infected bodily fluids being exchanged is minimal in most areas of everyday practice. Thus, in contrast to the emergency room scenario, the degree of contact between most therapists and their clients is roughly of the nature of social contact. In this connection, Smithurst argues that, on existing evidence, 'ordinary human intercourse, bar the sexual, is not a circumstance of very low risk of HIV infection, but one of no risk at all' (Smithurst, 1990:103). Consequently, while the trauma surgeon might well argue that the nature of his or her work creates a special need to know patients' HIV status – and a duty on the part of patients who know themselves to be infected to warn (Elder, 1989) – the average therapist can hardly claim a greater need to know than any member of the public who may come into social contact with an HIV-infected person.

Now, to say that the therapist has no more need to know than ordinary members of the public is not to say that the therapist has no need to know whatsoever. It might still be argued that knowledge of a client's HIV status will enable the therapist to protect him- or herself. It is doubtful, however, that this is the case, for a number of reasons.

First, it must be remembered that while a number of HIV-positive people know themselves to be such, a far greater number are undiagnosed. Therefore, knowing the HIV status of clients in this first category will be of no assistance in protecting the therapist from infection by those in the second category.

Second, although the fact that a person is seropositive is fairly good evidence that he or she has the virus, the converse does not necessarily apply to a person who has tested seronegative. Following inoculation with the virus, there is a period of anything up to six months (or even longer) before antibodies appear (Fan *et al.*, 1996), and during this period any test will be negative. Thus, a person tested on a given day may have been infected for several weeks or months prior to this test and still produce a negative result. Alternatively, on rare occasions an individual may be infected but never produce antibodies, and therefore always provide a false negative test.

Furthermore, even if the test is a true negative, this only tells us his or her HIV status at that time – it obviously does not guarantee that the individual has remained HIV-negative since the test. It follows from these observations that it is possible to identify only a small minority of those clients who are HIV-positive, and any precautions to prevent infection should therefore be taken in respect of *all* clients, not merely those known to be seropositive. The risk of the *procedure* forms the basis of these measures, not the risk thought to be posed by the individual *patient* (Mercier and Haig, 1993).

The precautions in question are the so-called 'universal precautions' recommended by bodies such as the Centers for Disease Control in the USA (reprinted in Pratt, 1995). These advocate the use of protective materials only when working with fluids such as blood and blood-derived fluids such as cerebrospinal and synovial fluids, or with other fluids that contain traces of blood. It is also recommended that any part of the body that comes into contact with potentially infectious bodily fluids should be washed immediately and thoroughly, and that health professionals with weeping skin lesions should avoid direct patient care. These are not very dramatic precautions; nor do they need to be, as HIV is relatively difficult to transmit. The virus survives for only a short time outside the human body, and is readily killed with routine disinfection procedures (Elder, 1989; Fan *et al.*, 1996). Even in the event of skin puncture with an infected object, the risk of transmission from a single such inoculation injury has been estimated at less than 0.4 per cent (Becker *et al.*, 1989; Jeffries, 1992), whereas the likelihood of contracting the hepatitis B virus through such an injury has been put at approximately 30 per cent (Pratt, 1995). This poses a far more substantial risk. Between 200 and 300 deaths occur annually among health care workers in the USA through hepatitis B (Gerberding, 1990); Pratt (1995) reports that the figure for occupational HIV infection, since the beginning of the epidemic, is approximately 100.

Accordingly, unless there is a likelihood of coming into contact with the client's blood or other potentially infectious bodily fluids – unlikely in the context of most areas of practice in therapy – there is no need to adopt special protective measures. Indeed, any such special measures taken in respect of clients known to be seropositive are likely to be counterproductive. If a special policy is adopted for known carriers of the virus, this may lead to a dangerous carelessness and complacency in respect of other patients assumed (in some cases falsely) to be 'safe'. Instead of implementing special measures for special cases, the most effective way to protect health care staff from infection with HIV or other pathogens is likely to be through institutional arrangements and practices which encourage and facilitate compliance with standard precautions (Tuohey, 1995).

These universal precautions, including protective measures where contact with blood is likely, should be taken routinely in respect of each and every patient; there is therefore no advantage to the therapist from knowledge of a given client's HIV status. Indeed, it should be remembered that, because of their immunocompromised condition, clients with HIV infection are likely to be at greater risk from the therapist than vice versa. This, in theory, would be a far more powerful argument for therapists to know their clients' HIV status. However, the practical disadvantages – in terms of unknown HIV carriers, and so forth – would be just the same.

Both of the arguments which might support the therapist's need to know clients' HIV status have been shown to be flawed. It was suggested in Chapter 5 that there is a presumption in favour of respecting privacy and confidentiality. It was further proposed that it is only when the consequences of observing privacy or confidentiality are sufficiently bad that the requirement to do so can be abrogated. It has yet to be demonstrated that such consequences are likely to follow if therapists are unaware of whether or not their clients are seropositive. In contrast, there are likely to be serious consequences of any relaxing of the requirements of confidentiality:

- Clients may be subject to discriminatory care within the health care system.
- If information is made known in the wider society, clients may face prejudice, stigma and discrimination in employment and social life, and in relation to life insurance.

• In the light of the above practices, those who feel they may be HIV-positive, or suspect they are experiencing the early symptoms of AIDS, may be reluctant to come forward for testing.

It would seem, therefore, that therapists have no real need to know the HIV status of their clients, as this has no real bearing on the interventions they may perform or the precautions that should be taken with respect to a particular client. However, another situation may arise regarding clients' HIV status which is less easy to resolve; the issue here is not whether the therapist should know, but, given that the therapist knows, whether this information can legitimately be passed on to a third party.

Should third parties be told?

Gillett (1987) describes a case in which a man presenting with a dry persistent cough and a history of night sweats is found to be HIV-positive. He admits to being an active bisexual. However, despite repeated persuasion, he refuses to allow the diagnosis to be conveyed to his wife, even though he continues to have an active sexual relationship with her. Some eighteen months later, shortly before his death from AIDS, he allows his wife to be told. She is tested and found to be seropositive; she later displays the early signs of AIDS.

Here, much the same arguments supporting confidentiality are at stake – the prima facie duty to preserve confidences as part of the fiduciary relationship between patient and practitioner, the danger of loss of trust if such confidences are routinely broken, and so forth. However, in a case such as this there are three reasons to think that it might nonetheless be permissible to breach the confidentiality requirement. First, the consequences of maintaining confidentiality are significantly more serious in this case. Arguably, secrecy on the part of the health professional has resulted in the wife's contracting a fatal disease which she might otherwise have prevented. Second, although there may not exist a direct professional relationship between the therapist and the wife, nonetheless considerations of beneficence suggest that the therapist should seek to protect her from a major avoidable harm. This can be weighed against the requirement, based on respect for autonomy, to respect the husband's wish for secrecy, and might be felt to be of greater priority. Finally, it can be argued, as Gillett (1987) does, that the husband's disregard of his wife's welfare may serve to annul the duty to maintain confidentiality. It is as if the husband's callousness towards his wife disqualifies him from the right to confidentiality which he would normally enjoy:

> In the face of an expressed disregard for the harm being caused to those others concerned, we will be morally correct in abandoning what would otherwise be a binding obligation. We should and do feel the need to preserve and protect the already affected life of the potential victim of his deception and in this feeling we exhibit a sensitivity to moral rectitude. (Gillett, 1987:19)

Gillett goes on to emphasize that disclosure must be restricted to those at risk of harm, and that there would be no justification for informing those who are not at such risk – for example, the husband's employers, friends, or other members of his family with whom he is not engaging in at-risk behaviour.

There would seem, therefore, to be a far stronger case for overriding the confidentiality requirement in the case of at-risk third parties than in respect of health professionals. However, this will only be justifiable where the third party concerned is at genuine risk of infection. It should also be recalled that, if viewed in consequentialist terms, the short-term benefits of breaching confidentiality in an individual case such as this must be weighed against the long-term harm that such a policy might cause (Gillon, 1987; Brazier and Lobjoit, 1990). Allmark (1995) points out that facilities such as genito-urinary medicine clinics and needle exchange centres for drug users would effectively be unable to operate if they were thought to offer less than complete confidentiality.

Who needs to know the therapist's HIV status?

A question which remains to be addressed is whether clients have a right to know the HIV status of those caring for them. If so, should health care workers undergo compulsory HIV testing? These are important questions, for whether or not they *need* to know, there is evidence that members of the public *want* to know the HIV status of those caring for them (Marshall *et al.*, 1990).

In relation to the first of these questions, the issues are much the same as in the case of the client's HIV status. Again, the principal consideration is whether or not the health care worker poses a threat to the client's welfare. According to Pratt (1995), there is only one documented instance of practitioner-to-client transmission – the case of David Acer, a dentist in Florida who is thought to have infected six patients (Ou *et al.*, 1992; Ciesielski *et al.*, 1994). Transmission from an infected health care worker might occur directly in the course of a procedure which involved an exchange of blood (such as a puncture wound during the performance of an invasive procedure). It might also occur indirectly, such as if a health professional were to infect an instrument which was then used on a patient (it is thought that David Acer may have infected his patients in this way).

If we return to the case of the emergency room surgeon discussed earlier, it is clear that just as the surgeon might be at risk of infection from HIV-infected patients, so these patients might be at risk from the surgeon if he or she were infected, though probably less so (Gostin, 1989). Patients, it might be argued, would have a very real *need* to know the surgeon's HIV status; this would form the basis of a *right* to know, and a corresponding duty on the surgeon to tell. The same would not apply, however, in the case of most therapists. Except possibly in techniques such as acupuncture, the likelihood of transmission during therapeutic procedures is almost non-existent. Considering that the risk of seroconversion after an invasive procedure by an HIV-positive surgeon has been put at between 2.4 and 24 per million (Strax, 1994), the corresponding figure for transmission from a therapist must be vanishingly small. In any case, the HIV-infected health professional is likely to be at greater risk than the patients whom he or she is treating (Erridge, 1996).

Given that patients and clients have no substantial need, and thus no right, to know therapists' HIV status, the question of compulsory HIV testing largely evaporates. Such a practice would anyway be subject to the practical difficulties associated with the HIV antibody test which have already been outlined. Gostin argues:

Physicians who are not at increased risk for HIV or those who do not perform seriously invasive procedures have no legal or ethical obligation to be tested; and there should be no duty on health care facilities to screen them routinely. (Gostin, 1989:35)

In the UK, the United Kingdom Central Council for Nursing, Midwifery and Health Visiting (UKCC) and the British Medical Association (BMA) have both rejected routine testing of staff. However, it is also stressed that health professionals who know themselves to be HIV-infected should seek counselling and advice as to safe practice (UKCC, 1993; BMA, 1993). This is only likely to occur if practitioners trust the confidentiality of such a process.

A question of values

The sorts of ethical issues we have been considering in respect of AIDS and HIV infection are complicated, and made all the more urgent by the negative perceptions and emotions which often surround this subject. Health professionals are not immune to the stereotyped and prejudiced views which are found in society at large. One of the most vivid expressions of such views was voiced early in the epidemic by a nurse in the UK:

[F]rankly, I have no sympathy with homosexuals who contract the disease. This is because it has been contracted through performing an unnatural act – a biological fact. Therefore, while nurses have a duty to care for the sick, we must also recognise that it is 'self-inflicted' in the truest sense of the term, and need not have arisen in the first place. What makes AIDS more horrific is that a stranger's perverse sexual actions can harm totally unknown innocents. (Napier, 1985)

A number of studies have disclosed varying degrees of fear, disgust and discrimination among health professionals and students (e.g. Kelly *et al.*, 1987; Royse and Birge, 1987; Atchison *et al.*, 1990). It is interesting to compare the reaction to the perceived dangers of HIV with earlier responses to hepatitis B. Bosk and Frader (1991) note that the hazards of contact with the hepatitis virus caused considerable discussion and debate in medical journals in the 1970s, and there was strong evidence of occupational inoculation and transmission. However, they point out that there was no suggestion of declining to treat infected patients. That such a suggestion is sometimes made today may reflect, at least partially, the very different moral connotations surrounding HIV infection.

Just as was noted in the earlier discussion of suicide, therapists may have strong personal views on issues associated with HIV infection and AIDS. However, it is important to consider when personal values and convictions are an appropriate determinant of professional care, and when they are not. Most would agree that feelings of compassion, sympathy, altruism and the like are important motivating factors within the therapy professions, and the idea that therapists should seek to achieve some form of absolute 'affective neutrality' is rather outdated. Nonetheless, it is recognized that certain values, if allowed to influence the conduct of professional practice, are likely to be inimical to the welfare of certain patients. Hence, there is a widespread view that health professionals should strive for a form of 'detached concern'. This has been defined in the following way:

> The process by which students gradually learn to combine the counter-attitudes of detachment and concern to attain the balance between objectivity and empathy expected of mature physicians in the various kinds of professional situations they encounter. (Fox, 1979:56)

Thus, whereas empathy and emotional rapport may be valuable in helping therapists to gain insight into the nature of clients' problems and to determine what might be appropriate and acceptable means of intervention, notions of approval or disapproval, like or dislike, or judgements of social worth, are likely to detract from high-quality professional care. It will be recalled from the discussion of different approaches to resource allocation in Chapter 7 that such value judgements are likely to be arbitrary at best, and discriminatory at worst.

Concluding remarks

This final chapter has explored a number of topics which are of considerable relevance to therapists, but which had not been addressed in detail in previous chapters. There are, of course, other such topics: if it were not for limitations of space, more could have been said about the ethical issues that arise in counselling, the care of comatose patients, the rehabilitation of children, record keeping, managing clients with learning difficulties, and so forth. However, it is hoped that this book will have equipped therapists with the necessary skills for them to examine these and other topics for themselves, and resolve some of the conflicts to which they give rise.

References

Ahorny, L. and Strasser, S. (1993). Patient satisfaction: what we know and what we still need to explore. *Medical Care Review*, **50**, 49-79.

Alderson, P. (1990). *Choosing for Children: Parents' Consent to Surgery*. Oxford: Oxford University Press.

Alderson, P. (1993). *Children's Consent to Surgery*. Buckingham: Open University Press.

Allmark, P. (1995). HIV and the boundaries of confidentiality. *Journal of Advanced Nursing*, **21**, 158-163.

Allmark, P. and Klarzynski, R. (1992). The case against nurse advocacy. *British Journal of Nursing*, **2**, 33-36.

Anonymous (1982). On telling dying patients the truth. *Journal of Medical Ethics*, **8**, 115-116.

Anscombe, G. E. M. (1958). Modern moral philosophy. *Philosophy*, **33**, 1-9.

AOTA (1989). Human immunodeficiency virus (position paper): American Occupational Therapy Association Commission on Practice. *American Journal of Occupational Therapy*, **43**, 803-804.

AOTA (1993). Core values and attitudes of occupational therapy practice: American Occupational Therapy Association Commission on Standards and Ethics. *American Journal of Occupational Therapy*, **47**, 1085-1086.

AOTA (1994). Occupational therapy code of ethics: American Occupational Therapy Association Commission on Standards and Ethics. *American Journal of Occupational Therapy*, **48**, 1037-1038.

AOTA (1996). Enforcement procedure for occupational therapy code of ethics: American Occupational Therapy Association Commission on Standards and Ethics. *American Journal of Occupational Therapy*, **50**, 848-852.

APA (1990). Australian Physiotherapy Association: Ethical Principles. *Australian Journal of Physiotherapy*, **36**, 117-121.

Appelbaum, P. S. and Grisso, T. (1988). Assessing patients' capacities to consent to treatment. *New England Journal of Medicine*, **319**, 1635-1638.

Appelbaum, P. S., Lidz, C. W. and Meisel, A. (1987). *Informed Consent: Legal Theory and Clinical Practice*. New York: Oxford University Press.

Appelbaum, P. S. and Roth, L. H. (1982). Competency to consent to research: a psychiatric overview. *Archives of General Psychiatry*, **39**, 951-958.

APTA (1991). *Code of Ethics*. Alexandria: American Physical Therapy Association.

APTA (1995). *Guide for Professional Conduct*. Alexandria: American Physical Therapy Association.

Atchison, B. J., Beard, B. J. and Lester, L. B. (1990). Occupational therapy personnel and AIDS: attitudes, knowledge, and fears. *American Journal of Occupational Therapy*, **44**, 212-217.

Bach, J. R. and Barnett, V. (1994). Ethical considerations in the management of individuals with severe neuromuscular disorders. *American Journal of Physical Medicine and Rehabilitation*, **73**, 134-140.

Bailey, D. M. and Schwartzberg, S. L. (1995). *Ethical and Legal Dilemmas in Occupational Therapy*, Philadelphia: W.B. Saunders.

Bakland, L. K., Burlew, S. A., Clements, M. J. *et al.* (1989). Health care professionals' role in the treatment of AIDS. In *AIDS and the Allied Health Professions* (J. W. Hopp and E. A. Rogers, eds), Philadelphia: F.A. Davis.

Baly, M. (1984). *Professional Responsibility*, 2nd edn. Chichester: John Wiley.

Banja, J. D. (1986). Proxy consent to medical treatment: implications for rehabilitation. *Archives of Physical Medicine and Rehabilitation*, **67**, 790-792.

Banks, S. (1995). *Ethics and Values in Social Work*. London: Macmillan.

BAOT (1990). *Code of Professional Conduct*. London: British Association of Occupational Therapists.

Barkes, P. (1979). Bioethics and informed consent in American health care delivery. *Journal of Advanced Nursing*, **4**, 23-38.

Barman, C. R. and Hendrix, J. R. (1983). Exploring bioethical issues: an instructional model. *American Biology Teacher*, **45**, 23-31.

Barnitt, R. (1993). What gives you sleepless nights? Ethical practice in occupational therapy. *British Journal of Occupational Therapy*, **56**, 207-212.

Barnitt, R. (1994). Truth telling in occupational therapy and physiotherapy. *British Journal of Occupational Therapy*, **57**, 334-340.

Barnitt, R. and Fulton, C. (1994). Patient agreement to treatment: a framework for therapists. *British Journal of Therapy and Rehabilitation*, **1**, 121-127.

Battin, M. P. (1994). *The Least Worst Death: Essays in Bioethics on the End of Life*. New York: Oxford University Press.

Beauchamp, T. L. (1989). A reply to Rachels on active and passive euthanasia. In *Cross Cultural Perspectives in Medical Ethics: A Reader* (R. M. Veatch, ed.), Boston: Jones and Bartlett.

Beauchamp, T. L. and Childress, J. F. (1994). *Principles of Biomedical Ethics*, 4th edn. New York: Oxford University Press.

Becker, C. E., Cone, J. E. and Gerberding, J. (1989). Occupational infection with human immunodeficiency virus (HIV): risks and risk reduction. *Annals of Internal Medicine*, **110**, 653–656.

Bell, N. K. (1992). If age becomes a standard for rationing health care... In *Feminist Perspectives in Medical Ethics* (H. B. Holmes and L. M. Purdy, eds), Bloomington: Indiana University Press.

Benjamin, M. and Curtis, J. (1986). *Ethics in Nursing*, 2nd edn. New York: Oxford University Press.

Benson, J. and Britten, N. (1996). Respecting the autonomy of cancer patients when talking with their families: qualitative analysis of semistructured interviews with patients. *British Medical Journal*, **313**, 729–731.

Bernal, E. W. (1992). The nurse as patient advocate. *Hastings Center Report*, **22**, 18–23.

Bird, A. W. (1994). Enhancing patient well-being: advocacy or negotiation? *Journal of Medical Ethics*, **20**, 152–156.

BMA (1993). *Medical Ethics Today: Its Practice and Philosophy*. London: British Medical Association.

Bok, S. (1978). *Lying: Moral Choice in Public and Private Life*. Hassocks: Harvester Press.

Bok, S. (1984). *Secrets: On the Ethics of Concealment and Revelation*. Oxford: Oxford University Press.

Bosk, C. L. and Frader, J. E. (1991). AIDS and its impact on medical work. In *A Disease of Society: Cultural and Institutional Responses to AIDS* (D. Nelkin, D. P. Willis and S. V. Parris, eds), Cambridge: Cambridge University Press.

Brandstetter, R. D. (1992). Intensive care for the elderly: should the gates remain open? *New York State Journal of Medicine*, **92**, 175–176.

Brazier, M. (1992). *Medicine, Patients and the Law*, 2nd edn. Harmondsworth: Penguin Books.

Brazier, M. and Lobjoit, M. (1990). AIDS, ethics, and the respiratory physician. *Thorax*, **45**, 283–286.

Brewin, T. B. (1985). Truth, trust, and paternalism. *Lancet*, **2**, 490–491.

Brewin, T. B. (1993). How much ethics is needed to make a good doctor? *Lancet*, **341**, 161–163.

Brock, D. W. (1989). Death and dying. In *Medical Ethics: An Introduction* (R. M. Veatch, ed.), Boston: Jones and Bartlett.

Brock, D. W. (1993). *Life and Death: Philosophical Essays in Biomedical Ethics.* Cambridge: Cambridge University Press.

Brown, J. M., Kitson, A. L. and McKnight, T. J. (1992). *Challenges in Caring: Explorations in Nursing and Ethics.* London: Chapman & Hall.

Bruce-Jones, P. (1996). Resuscitation decisions in the elderly: a discussion of current thinking. *Journal of Medical Ethics*, **22**, 286–291.

Bruce-Jones, P., Roberts, H., Bowker, L. and Cooney, V. (1996). Resuscitating the elderly: what do the patients want? *Journal of Medical Ethics*, **22**, 154–159.

Bruckner, J. (1987). Physical therapists as double agents: ethical dilemmas of divided loyalties. *Physical Therapy*, **67**, 383–387.

Buchanan, A. (1989). Health-care delivery and resource allocation. In *Medical Ethics* (R. M. Veatch, ed.), Boston: Jones and Bartlett.

Buchanan, A. E. and Brock, D. W. (1989). *Deciding for Others: the Ethics of Surrogate Decision Making.* Cambridge: Cambridge University Press.

Buckman, R. (1992). *How to Break Bad News: A Guide for Health-Care Professionals.* London: Papermac.

Bytheway, B. and Johnson, J. (1990). On defining ageism. *Critical Social Policy*, **10**, 27–39.

Callahan, D. (1991). Limiting health care for the old. In *Aging and Ethics: Philosophical Problems in Gerontology* (N. S. Jecker, ed.), Totowa: Humana Press.

Callahan, D. (1995). Allocating health care resources: the vexing case of rehabilitation. *American Journal of Physical Medicine and Rehabilitation*, **74** (suppl.), S7–S11.

Callahan, J. C. (1988). Basics and background. In *Ethical Issues in Professional Life* (J. C. Callahan, ed.), New York: Oxford University Press.

Campbell, A. (1984). *Moderated Love: A Theology of Professional Care.* London: SPCK.

Campbell, A., Gillett, G. and Jones, G. (1992). *Practical Medical Ethics.* Auckland: Oxford University Press.

Campbell, T. (1988). *Justice.* London: Macmillan.

Caplan, A. L. (1988). Informed consent and provider–patient relationships in rehabilitation medicine. *Archives of Physical Medicine and Rehabilitation*, **69**, 312–317.

Caplan, A. L. (1992). Ethics, cost-containment, and the allocation of scarce resources. In *If I was a Rich Man Could I buy a Pancreas?*

And other Essays on the Ethics of Health Care (A. L. Caplan), Bloomington: Indiana University Press.

Capron, A. M. (1974). Informed consent in catastrophic disease research and treatment. *University of Pennsylvania Law Review*, **123**, 340–438.

Capron, A. M. (1986). Legal and ethical problems in decisions for death. *Law, Medicine and Health Care*, **14**, 141–144.

Cassidy, J. C. (1988). Access to health care: a clinician's opinion about an ethical issue. *American Journal of Occupational Therapy*, **42**, 295–299.

Childress, J. F. (1982). *Who Should Decide? Paternalism in Health Care*. NewYork: Oxford University Press.

Ciesielski, C. A., Marianos, D. W., Schochetman, G. *et al.* (1994). The 1990 Florida dental investigation: the press and the science. *Annals of Internal Medicine*, **121**, 886–888.

Clawson, A. L. (1994). The relationship between clinical decision making and ethical decision making. *Physiotherapy*, **80**, 10–14.

Coates, R. (1990a). HIV infection and AIDS: a guide for physiotherapists. *Australian Journal of Physiotherapy*, **36**, 17–21.

Coates, R. (1990b). Ethics and physiotherapy. *Australian Journal of Physiotherapy*, **36**, 84–87.

Collins, J. (1988). Should doctors tell the truth? In *Ethical Issues in Professional Life* (J. C. Callahan, ed.), New York: Oxford University Press.

Cooper, M. H. (1975). *Rationing Health Care*. London: Croom Helm.

Copp, L. A. (1986). The nurse as advocate for vulnerable persons. *Journal of Advanced Nursing*, **11**, 255–263.

Corr, C. A. and Corr, D. M. (1986). Developing a philosophy for caring. In *Cash's Textbook of Neurology for Physiotherapists*, 4th edn (P. A. Downie, ed.), London: Faber and Faber.

COT (1993). *Statement on Consent for Occupational Therapy*, (SPP 195). London: College of Occupational Therapists.

COT (1995). *Code of Ethics and Professional Conduct for Occupational Therapists*. London: College of Occupational Therapists.

Cousins, N. (1980). A layman looks at truth telling in medicine. *Journal of the American Medical Association*, **244**, 1929–1930.

Coy, J. A. (1989a). Autonomy-based informed consent: Ethical implications for patient noncompliance. *Physical Therapy*, **69**, 826–833.

Coy, J. A. (1989b). Philosophic aspects of patient noncompliance: a critical analysis. *Topics in Geriatric Rehabilitation*, **4**, 52–60.

CPA (1989). *Code of Ethics and Rules of Conduct*. Toronto: Canadian Physiotherapy Association.

CSP (1996a). *Rationing of Physiotherapy Services* (Information Paper PA 30). London: Chartered Society of Physiotherapy.

CSP (1996b). *Rules of Professional Conduct*. London: Chartered Society of Physiotherapy.

CST (1988). *Code of Ethics and Professional Conduct, with Ethical Guidelines for Research*. London: College of Speech Therapists.

Curtin, L. and Flaherty, M. J. (1982). *Nursing Ethics: Theories and Pragmatics*. Bowie: Robert J. Brady Co.

Cusack, L. and Singh, S. (1994). *HIV and AIDS Care: Practical Approaches*. London: Chapman & Hall.

Daniels, N (1985). *Just Health Care*. Cambridge: Cambridge University Press.

Delany, C. (1996). Should I warn the patient first? *Australian Journal of Physiotherapy*, **42**, 249-255.

Dike, L. (1993). Physiotherapists' perceptions of risk of HIV transmission in clinical practice. *Physiotherapy*, **79**, 178-185.

Dimond, B. (1995). *Legal Aspects of Nursing*, 2nd edn. London: Prentice Hall.

Dougherty, C. J. (1994). Quality-adjusted life years and the ethical values of health care. *American Journal of Physical Medicine and Rehabilitation*, **73**, 61-65.

Dougherty, C. J. and Purtilo, R. (1995), Physicians' duty of compassion. *Cambridge Quarterly of Healthcare Ethics*, **4**, 426-433.

Downie, R. S. and Calman, K. C. (1994). *Healthy Respect: Ethics in Health Care*, 2nd Edn. Oxford: Oxford University Press.

Downie, R. S. and Telfer, E. (1969). *Respect for Persons*. London: George Allen & Unwin.

Downie, R. S. and Telfer, E. (1980). *Caring and Curing: A Philosophy of Medicine and Social Work*. London: Methuen.

Doyal, L. (1995). Needs, rights, and equity: moral quality in healthcare rationing. *Quality in Health Care*, **4**, 273-283.

Drane, J. F. (1991). The many faces of competency. In *Biomedical Ethics*, 3rd edn (T. A. Mappes and J. S. Zembaty, eds), New York: McGraw-Hill.

Dresser, R. (1984). Bound to treatment: the Ulysses contract. *Hastings Center Report*, **14**, 13-16.

Drickamer, M. A. and Lachs, M. S. (1992). Should patients with Alzheimer's disease be told their diagnosis? *New England Journal of Medicine*, **326**, 947-951.

Dworkin, G. (1972). Paternalism. *Monist*, **56**, 64-84.

Dworkin, G. (1988). *The Theory and Practice of Autonomy*. Cambridge: Cambridge University Press.

Edgar, A. (1994). The value of codes of conduct. In *Ethical Issues in Nursing* (G. Hunt, ed.), London: Routledge.

Edwards, S. D. (1996). *Nursing Ethics: A Principle-Based Approach*. London: Macmillan.

Elder, H. A. (1989). Transmission of HIV and prevention of AIDS. In *AIDS and the Allied Health Professions* (J. W. Hopp and E. A. Rogers, eds), Philadelphia: F.A. Davis.

Ellin, J. S. (1982). Special professional morality and the duty of veracity. *Business and Professional Ethics Journal*, 1, 75-90.

Ellos, W. J. (1990). *Ethical Practice in Clinical Medicine*. London: Routledge.

Emanuel, E. J., Fairclough, D. L., Daniels, E. R. and Clarridge, B. R. (1996). Euthanasia and physician-assisted suicide: attitudes and experiences of oncology patients, oncologists, and the public. *Lancet*, 347, 1805-1810.

Emery, D. D. and Schneiderman, L. J. (1989). Cost-effectiveness analysis in health care. *Hastings Center Report*, 19, 8-13.

Engelhardt, H. T. Jr (1986). *The Foundations of Bioethics*. New York: Oxford University Press.

Engelhardt, H. T. Jr (1991). Rights to health care: created, not discovered. In *Rights to Health Care* (T. J. Bole and W. B. Bondeson, eds), Dordrecht: Kluwer Academic Publishers.

Erridge, P. (1996). The rights of HIV infected healthcare workers. *British Medical Journal*, 312, 1625-1626.

Evans, R. W., Manninen, D. L., Garrison, L. P. Jr, *et al.* (1985). The quality of life of patients with end-stage renal failure. *New England Journal of Medicine*, 312, 553-559.

Faden, R. F. and Beauchamp, T. L. (1986). *A History and Theory of Informed Consent*. New York: Oxford University Press.

Fairbairn, G. J. (1995). *Contemplating Suicide: The Language and Ethics of Self Harm*. London: Routledge.

Falk-Kessler, J., Barnowski, C. and Salvant, S. (1994). Mandatory HIV testing and occupational therapists. *American Journal of Occupational Therapy*, 48, 27-37.

Fan, H., Conner, R. F. and Villarreal, L. P. (1996). *AIDS: Science and Society*. Boston: Jones and Bartlett.

Faulder, C. (1985). *Whose Body Is It? The Troubling Issue of Informed Consent*. London: Virago.

Fletcher, N., Holt, J., Brazier, M. and Harris, J. (1995). *Ethics, Law and Nursing*. Manchester: Manchester University Press.

Fortinsky, R. H. (1993). How much rehabilitation potential is in long-term care? Using data for informed practice. *Topics in Geriatric Rehabilitation*, 9, 1-10.

Fox, R. C. (1979). The autopsy: its place in the attitude-learning of second-year medical students. In *Essays in Medical Sociology: Journeys into the Field* (R. C. Fox, ed.), New York: John Wiley.

Frankena, W. K. (1963). *Ethics*. Englewood Cliffs: Prentice-Hall.

Freidson, E. (1970). *Profession of Medicine: A Study of the Sociology of Applied Knowledge*. New York: Dodd, Mead & Company.

French, S. (1994). The disabled role. In *On Equal Terms: Working with Disabled People* (S. French, ed.), Oxford: Butterworth-Heinemann.

French, S. (1997). Ageism. In *Physiotherapy: A Psychosocial Approach*, 2nd edn. (S. French, ed.), Oxford: Butterworth-Heinemann.

Fromer, M. J. (1981). *Ethical Issues in Health Care*. St Louis: C.V. Mosby.

Gallaher, E. B. (1976). Lines of reconstruction and extension in the Parsonian sociology of illness. *Social Science and Medicine*, **10**, 207-218.

Garnham, J. C. (1975). Some observations on informed consent in non-therapeutic research. *Journal of Medical Ethics*, **1**, 138-145.

Gates, B. (1994). *Advocacy: A Nurses' Guide*. London: Scutari Press.

Gerberding, J. L. (1990). Current epidemiologic evidence and case reports of occupationally acquired HIV and other bloodborne diseases. *Infection Control and Hospital Epidemiology*, **11**, 558-560.

Gerberding, J. L., Littell, C., Tarkington, A. *et al.* (1990). Risk of exposure of surgical personnel to patients' blood during surgery at San Francisco General Hospital. *New England Journal of Medicine*, **322**, 1788-1793.

Gillett, G. (1987). AIDS and confidentiality. *Journal of Applied Philosophy*, **4**, 15-20.

Gillon, R. (1986). *Philosophical Medical Ethics*. Chichester: John Wiley.

Gillon, R. (1987). AIDS and medical confidentiality. *British Medical Journal*, **294**, 1675-1677.

Gillon, R. (1994a). The four principles revisited – a reappraisal. In *Principles of Health Care Ethics* (R. Gillon and A. Lloyd, eds), Chichester: John Wiley.

Gillon, R. (1994b). Medical ethics: four principles plus attention to scope. *British Medical Journal*, **309**, 184-188.

Gitlin, L. N. (1993). Therapeutic dilemmas in the care of the elderly in rehabilitation. *Topics in Geriatric Rehabilitation*, **9**, 11-20.

Glover, J. (1977). *Causing Death and Saving Lives*. Harmondsworth: Penguin Books.

Goldie, L. (1982). The ethics of telling the patient. *Journal of Medical Ethics*, **8**, 128-133.

Gostin, L. (1989). HIV-infected physicians and the practice of seriously invasive procedures. *Hastings Center Report*, **19**, 32–39.

Guccione, A. A. (1980). Ethical issues in physical therapy practice: a survey of physical therapists in New England. *Physical Therapy*, **60**, 1264–1272.

Guccione, A. A. (1988a). Compliance and patient autonomy: ethical and legal limits to professional dominance. *Topics in Geriatric Rehabilitation*, **3**, 62–73.

Guccione, A .A. (1988b). Needs of the elderly and the politics of health care. *Physical Therapy*, **68**, 1386–1390.

Guthrie, D. J. (1957). The Hippocratic Oath. In *Medical Ethics: A Guide to Students and Practitioners* (M. Davidson, ed.), London: Lloyd-Luke.

Hailstone, J. D. (1969). The importance of the relationship between physiotherapist and patient. *Physiotherapy*, **55**, 230–232.

Hansen, R. A. (1988). Ethics is the issue. *American Journal of Occupational Therapy*, **42**, 279–281.

Hansen, R. A. (1990). The ethics of caring for patients with AIDS. *American Journal of Occupational Therapy*, **44**, 239–242.

Hare, R. M. (1981). *Moral Thinking: Its Levels, Method and Point.* Oxford: Clarendon Press.

Harris, J. (1985). *The Value of Life: An Introduction to Medical Ethics.* London: Routledge & Kegan Paul.

Harris, J. (1987). QALYfying the value of life. *Journal of Medical Ethics*, **13**, 117–123.

Harris, J. (1988). More and better justice. In *Philosophy and Medical Welfare* (J. M. Bell and S. Mendus, eds), Cambridge, Cambridge University Press.

Hart, E. and Bond, M. (1995). *Action Research for Health and Social Care: A Guide to Practice.* Buckingham: Open University Press.

Heyd, D. and Bloch, S. (1991). The ethics of suicide. In *Psychiatric Ethics*, 2nd edn (S. Bloch and P. Chodoff, eds), Oxford: Oxford University Press.

Higgs, R. (1994). Truth-telling, lying and the doctor–patient relationship. In *Principles of Health Care Ethics* (R. Gillon and A.Lloyd, eds), Chichester: John Wiley.

Holm, S. (1993). What is wrong with compliance? *Journal of Medical Ethics*, **19**, 108–110.

Hopkins, A., Gabbay, J. and Neuberger, J. (1994) Role of users of health care in achieving a quality service. *Quality in Health Care*, **3**, 203–209.

Howard, B. S. (1991). How high do we jump? The effect of reimbursement on occupational therapy. *American Journal of Occupational Therapy*, **45**, 875–881.

Hunt, G. (1992). What is nursing ethics? *Nurse Education Today*, **12**, 323–328.

Hunt, G. (1995). *Whistleblowing in the Health Service: Accountability, Law and Professional Practice*. London: Edward Arnold.

Hunt, R. W. (1993). A critique of using age to ration health care. *Journal of Medical Ethics*, **19**, 19–23.

Hussey, T. (1996). Nursing ethics and professional codes of conduct. *Nursing Ethics*, **3**, 250–258.

Ingelfinger, F. J. (1972). Informed (but uneducated) consent. *New England Journal of Medicine*, **287**, 465–466.

Ingelfinger, F. J. (1980). Arrogance. *New England Journal of Medicine*, **303**, 1507–1511.

Jackson, J. (1992). Against killing the patient. In *Philosophy and Health Care* (E. Matthews and M. Menlowe, eds), Aldershot: Avebury.

Jackson, J. (1994). Promise-keeping and the doctor–patient relationship. In *Principles of Health Care Ethics* (R. Gillon and A. Lloyd, eds), Chichester: John Wiley.

Jecker, N. S. and Schneiderman, L. J. (1992) Futility and rationing. *American Journal of Medicine*, **92**, 189–196.

Jeffreys, M. (1993). Geriatric medicine: some ethical issues associated with its development. In *Choices and Decisions in Health Care* (A. Grubb, ed.), Chichester: John Wiley.

Jeffries, D. J. (1992). Doctors, patients, and HIV. *British Medical Journal*, **304**, 1258–1259.

Jennett, B. (1986). *High Technology Medicine: Benefits and Burdens*. Oxford: Oxford University Press.

Jette, A. M. and Bottomley, J. M. (1987). The graying of America: opportunities for physical therapy. *Physical Therapy*, **67**, 1537–1542.

Johnstone, M.-J. (1994). *Bioethics: A Nursing Perspective*, 2nd edn. Sydney: W.B. Saunders/Baillière Tindall.

Kasting, G. A. (1994). The nonnecessity of euthanasia. In *Biomedical Ethics Reviews 1993: Physician-Assisted Death* (J. M. Humber, R. F. Almeder and G. A. Kasting, eds), Totowa: Humana Press.

Kelly, J. A., St Lawrence, J. S., Smith, S. *et al.* (1987). Medical students' attitudes toward AIDS and homosexual patients. *Journal of Medical Education*, **62**, 549–556.

Kelner, M. (1995). Activists and delegators: elderly patients' preferences about control at the end of life. *Social Science and Medicine*, **41**, 537–545.

Klassen, A., Fitzpatrick, R., Jenkinson, C. and Goodacre, T. (1996). Should breast reduction surgery be rationed? A comparison of the health status of patients before and after treatment: postal questionnaire survey. *British Medical Journal*, **313**, 454–457.

Knibbs, J. (1993). Behaviour therapy. In *Childhood Onset Anorexia Nervosa and Related Eating Disorders* (B. Lask and R. Bryant-Waugh, eds), Hove: Lawrence Erlbaum Associates.

Koehn, D. (1994). *The Ground of Professional Ethics*. London: Routledge.

Kottow, M. H. (1986). Medical confidentiality: an intransigent and absolute obligation. *Journal of Medical Ethics*, **12**, 117–122.

Kottow, M. H. (1994). Stringent and predictable medical confidentiality. In *Principles of Health Care Ethics* (R. Gillon and A. Lloyd, eds), Chichester: John Wiley.

Kuhse, H. (1984). A modern myth. That letting die is not the intentional causation of death: some reflections on the trial and acquittal of Dr Leonard Arthur. *Journal of Applied Philosophy*, **1**, 21–38.

Kyler-Hutchison, P. (1988). Ethical reasoning and informed consent in occupational therapy. *American Journal of Occupational Therapy*, **42**, 283–287.

Lamb, D. (1988). *Down the Slippery Slope: Arguing in Applied Ethics*. London: Croom Helm.

Lamb, D. (1990). *Organ Transplants and Ethics*. Routledge: London.

Latourette, A. W. (1992). Right to privacy vs. right to know. *Clinical Management*, **12**, 54–61.

Lesser, H. (1991). The patient's right to information. In *Protecting the Vulnerable: Autonomy and Consent in Health Care* (M. Brazier and M. Lobjoit, eds), London: Routledge.

Lewis, C. B. and Bottomley, J. M. (1994) *Geriatric Physical Therapy: A Clinical Approach*. Norwalk: Appleton & Lange.

Loewy, E. H. (1989). *Textbook of Medical Ethics*. New York: Plenum Medical Book Company.

Loewy, E. H. (1991). Involving patients in Do Not Resuscitate (DNR) decisions: an old issue raising its ugly head. *Journal of Medical Ethics*, **17**, 156–160.

McAteer, M. (1997). Death, dying and bereavement. In *Physiotherapy: A Psychosocial Approach*, 2nd edn. (S. French, ed.), Oxford: Butterworth-Heinemann.

McKinlay, J. B. (1975). Who is really ignorant – physician or patient? *Journal of Health and Social Behavior*, **16**, 3–11.

Macklin, R. (1982). The geriatric patient: ethical issues in care and treatment. In *Value Conflicts in Health Care Delivery* (B. Gruzalski and C. Nelson, eds), Cambridge: Ballinger Publishing.

MacLaren, J.-A. (1996). Rehabilitation through advocacy and empowerment. *British Journal of Therapy and Rehabilitation*, **3**, 492–497.

McLean, S. and Maher, G (1983). *Medicine, Morals and the Law*. Aldershot: Gower.

McNaughton, D. (1988). *Moral Vision: An Introduction to Ethics*. Oxford: Blackwell.

Maguire, C. P., Kirby, M., Coen, R. *et al.* (1996). Family members' attitudes toward telling the patient with Alzheimer's disease their diagnosis. *British Medical Journal*, **313**, 529–530.

Marshall, P. A., O'Keefe, J. P., Fisher, S. G. *et al.* (1990) Patients' fear of contracting acquired immunodeficiency syndrome from physicians. *Archives of Internal Medicine*, **150**, 1501–1506.

Mason, J. K. and McCall Smith, R. A. (1994). *Law and Medical Ethics*, 4th edn. London: Butterworths.

Melia, K. (1989). *Everyday Nursing Ethics*. London: Macmillan.

Mercier, C. and Haig, L. (1993). Infection control in physiotherapy. *Physiotherapy*, **79**, 385–387.

Miller, R. (1991). The ethics of involuntary commitment to mental health treatment. In *Psychiatric Ethics*, 2nd edn (S. Bloch and P. Chodoff, eds), Oxford: Oxford University Press.

Morris, J. (1994). Prejudice. In *On Equal Terms: Working with Disabled People* (S. French, ed.), Oxford: Butterworth-Heinemann.

Muir Gray, J. A. (1994). The health care of the elderly. In *Principles of Health Care Ethics* (R. Gillon and A. Lloyd, eds), Chichester: John Wiley.

Murphy, E. (1988). Psychiatric implications. In *Consent and the Incompetent Patient: Ethics, Law, and Medicine* (S. R. Hirsch and J. Harris, eds), London: Gaskell.

Naidoo, J. and Wills, J (1994). *Health Promotion: Foundations for Practice*. London: Baillière Tindall.

Napier, B. (1985). Assurances over AIDS are misleading and health staff should be cautious (letter). *Nursing Mirror*, **161**, 11.

Nau, J.-Y. (1996). La pandémie de sida progresse rapidement dans le tiers-monde. *Le Monde*, 7–8 July, 2.

Neuhaus, B. E. (1988). Ethical considerations in clinical reasoning: the impact of technology and cost containment. *American Journal of Occupational Therapy*, **42**, 288–294.

Newton, L. H. (1981). Lawgiving for professional life: reflections on the place of the professional code. *Business and Professional Ethics Journal*, **1**, 41–53.

Nicholson, R. H. (1994). Limitations of the four principles. In *Principles of Health Care Ethics* (R. Gillon and A. Lloyd, eds), Chichester: John Wiley.

Noddings, N. (1984). *Caring: a Feminine Approach to Ethics and Moral Education*. Berkeley: University of California Press.

Novack, D. H., Plumer, R., Smith, R. L. *et al*. (1979). Changes in physicians' attitudes toward telling the cancer patient. *Journal of the American Medical Association*, **241**, 897–900.

Oken, D. (1961). What to tell cancer patients. *Journal of the American Medical Association*, **175**, 1120–1128.

Ost, D. E. (1984). The 'right' not to know. *Journal of Medicine and Philosophy*, **9**, 301–312.

Ou, C.-Y., Ciesielski, C. A., Myers, G. *et al*. (1992). Molecular epidemiology of HIV transmission in a dental practice. *Science*, **256**, 1165–1171.

Øvretveit, J. (1985). Medical dominance and the development of professional autonomy in physiotherapy. *Sociology of Health and Illness*, **7**, 76–93.

Parsons, T. (1951). *The Social System*. London: Routledge & Kegan Paul.

Parsons, T. (1972). Definitions of health and illness in the light of American values and social structure. In *Patients, Physicians and Illness*, 2nd edn (E. G. Jaco, ed.), New York: Free Press.

Paton, H. J. (1958). *The Categorical Imperative: A Study in Kant's Moral Philosophy*, 3rd edn. London: Hutchinson.

Pellegrino, E. D. (1979). Toward a reconstruction of medical morality: the primacy of the act of profession and the fact of illness. *Journal of Medicine and Philosophy*, **4**, 32–56.

Pellegrino, E. D. and Thomasma, D. C. (1988). *For the Patient's Good: The Restoration of Beneficence in Health Care*. New York: Oxford University Press.

Pratt L., Seligmann, A. and Reader, G. W. (1957). Physicians' views on the level of medical information among patients. *American Journal of Public Health*, **47**, 1277–1283.

Pratt, R. (1995). *HIV and AIDS: A Strategy for Nursing Care*. London: Edward Arnold.

Purtilo, R. B. (1977). The American Physical Therapy Association's Code of Ethics. *Physical Therapy*, **57**, 1001–1006.

Purtilo, R. B. (1984). Applying the principles of informed consent to patient care: legal and ethical considerations for physical therapy. *Physical Therapy*, **64**, 934-937.

Purtilo, R. (1986). Professional responsibility in physiotherapy: old dimensions and new directions. *Physiotherapy*, **72**, 579-583.

Purtilo, R. (1987a). Codes of ethics in physiotherapy: a retrospective view and look ahead. *Physiotherapy Practice*, **3**, 28-34.

Purtilo, R. B. (1987b). Ethical considerations. In *Therapeutic Considerations for the Elderly* (O. L. Jackson, ed.), New York: Churchill Livingstone.

Purtilo, R. B. (1988). Saying 'No' to patients for cost-related reasons: alternatives for the physical therapist. *Physical Therapy*, **68**, 1243-1247.

Purtilo, R. B. (1989). Ethical considerations in physical therapy. In *Physical Therapy* (R. M. Scully and M. R. Barnes, eds), Philadelphia: J.B. Lippincott.

Purtilo, R. B. (1993). *Ethical Dimensions in the Health Professions*, 2nd edn. Philadelphia: W.B. Saunders.

Purtilo, R. B. and Meier, R. H. (1995). Team challenges: regulatory constraints and patient empowerment. *American Journal of Physical Medicine and Rehabilitation*, **74** (Suppl.), S21-S24.

Rachels, J. (1975). Active and passive euthanasia. *New England Journal of Medicine*, **292**, 78-80.

Rachels, J. (1986). *The End of Life: Euthanasia and Morality*. Oxford: Oxford University Press.

Rachels, J. (1993). *The Elements of Moral Philosophy*, 2nd edn. New York: McGraw-Hill.

Raphael, D. D. (1967). Human rights, old and new. In *Political Theory and the Rights of Man* (D. D. Raphael, ed.), London: Macmillan.

Rawls, J. (1972). *A Theory of Justice*. Oxford: Oxford University Press.

Reed, K. L. and Sanderson, S. N. (1992). *Concepts of Occupational Therapy*, 2nd edn. Baltimore: Williams & Wilkins.

Richardson, J. (1992). Cost-utility analyses in health care: present status and future issues. In *Researching Health Care: Designs, Dilemmas, Disciplines* (J. Daly, I. McDonald and E. Willis, eds), London: Routledge.

Rigge, M. (1994). Involving patients in clinical audit. *Quality in Health Care*, **3** (Suppl.), S2-S5.

Ringel, E. (1980). Suicide prevention and the value of human life. In *Suicide: the Philosophical Issues* (M. P. Battin and D. Mayo, eds), New York: St Martin's Press.

Rivlin, M. M. (1995). Protecting elderly people: flaws in ageist arguments. *British Medical Journal*, **310**, 1179-1182.

Roberson, M. H. B. (1992). The meaning of compliance: patient perspectives. *Qualitative Health Research*, **2**, 7-26.

Robinson, J. A. T. (1973). The patient's right to know the truth. *Proceedings of the Royal Society of Medicine*, **66**, 536-537.

Ross, W. D. (1930). *The Right and the Good*. Oxford: Clarendon Press.

Roth, L. H., Meisel, A and Lidz, C. W. (1977). Tests of competency to consent to treatment. *American Journal of Psychiatry*, **134**, 279-284.

Royse, D. and Birge, B. (1987). Homophobia and attitudes towards AIDS patients among medical, nursing and paramedical students. *Psychological Reports*, **61**, 867-870.

Rumbold, G. (1993). *Ethics in Nursing Practice*, 2nd edn. London: Baillière Tindall.

Sade, R. M. (1971). Medical care as a right: a refutation. *New England Journal of Medicine*, **285**, 1288-1292.

Schade, S. G. and Muslin, H. (1989). Do not resuscitate decisions: discussions with patients. *Journal of Medical Ethics*, **15**, 186-190.

Schröck, R. (1980). A question of honesty in nursing practice. *Journal of Advanced Nursing*, **5**, 135-148.

Scofield, G. R. (1991). Is consent useful when resuscitation isn't? *Hastings Center Report*, **21**, 28-36.

Scofield. G. R. (1993). Ethical considerations in rehabilitation medicine. *Archives of Physical Medicine and Rehabilitation*, **74**, 341-346.

Seedhouse, D. (1986). *Health: the Foundations for Achievement*. Chichester: John Wiley.

Shaw, A. B. (1994). In defence of ageism. *Journal of Medical Ethics*, **20**, 188-191, 194.

Sheehan, J. (1985). Ethical considerations in nursing practice. *Journal of Advanced Nursing*, **10**, 331-336.

Sher, G. (1987). *Desert*. Princeton: Princeton University Press.

Sherwin, S. (1992). *No Longer Patient: Feminist Ethics and Health Care*. Temple University Press: Philadelphia.

Sidgwick, H. (1907). *The Methods of Ethics*, 7th edn. London: Macmillan.

Sieber, J. E. (1992). *Planning Ethically Responsible Research: A Guide for Students and Internal Review Boards*. Newbury Park: Sage Publications.

Siegler, M. (1991). Confidentiality in medicine - a decrepit concept. In *Biomedical Ethics*, 3rd edn (T. A. Mappes and J. S. Zembaty, eds), New York: McGraw-Hill.

Sikora, R. I. (1993). Rule utilitarianism and applied ethics. In *Applied*

Ethics: A Reader (E. R. Winkler and J. R. Coombs, eds), Oxford: Blackwell.

Sim, J. (1985). Physiotherapy: a professional profile. *Physiotherapy Practice*, **1**, 14-22.

Sim, J. (1986a). Truthfulness in the therapeutic relationship. *Physiotherapy Practice*, **2**, 121-127.

Sim, J. (1986b). Informed consent: ethical implications for physiotherapy. *Physiotherapy*, **72**, 584-587.

Sim, J. (1990). The concept of health. *Physiotherapy*, **76**, 423-428.

Sim, J. (1992). AIDS, nursing and occupational risk: an ethical analysis. *Journal of Advanced Nursing*, **17**, 569-575.

Sim, J. (1995). Moral rights and the ethics of nursing. *Nursing Ethics*, **2**, 31-40.

Sim, J. (1996a). Informed consent and manual therapy. *Manual Therapy*, **2**, 104-106.

Sim, J. (1996b). Client confidentiality: ethical issues in occupational therapy. *British Journal of Occupational Therapy*, **59**, 56-61.

Sim, J. and Purtilo, R. B. (1991). An ethical analysis of physical therapists' duty to treat persons with AIDS: Homosexual patients as a test case. *Physical Therapy*, **71**, 650-655.

Singleton, J. and McLaren, S. (1995). *Ethical Foundations of Health Care: Responsibilities in Decision Making*. London: Mosby.

Smithurst, M. (1990). AIDS: risks and discrimination. In *AIDS: A Moral Issue* (B. Almond, ed). Basingstoke: Macmillan.

Stimson, G. V. (1974). Obeying doctor's orders: a view from the other side. *Social Science and Medicine*, **8**, 97-104.

Stocker, M. (1976). The schizophrenia of modern moral theories. *Journal of Philosophy*, **73**, 453-466.

Strasser, M. (1986). Mill and the right to remain uninformed. *Journal of Medicine and Philosophy*, **11**, 265-278.

Strax, T. E. (1994). Ethical issues of treating patients with AIDS in a rehabilitation setting. *American Journal of Physical Medicine and Rehabilitation*, **73**, 293-295.

Strong, C. (1979). Informed consent: theory and policy. *Journal of Medical Ethics*, **5**, 196-199.

Styron, W. (1980). *Sophie's Choice*. New York: Bantam Books.

Sugarman, J. (1994). Hawkeye Pierce and the questionable relevance of medical etiquette to contemporary medical ethics and practice. *Journal of Clinical Ethics*, **5**, 224-230.

Sullivan, T. D. (1991). Active and passive euthanasia: an impertinent distinction? In *Biomedical Ethics*, 3rd edn (T. A. Mappes and J. S. Zembaty, eds), New York: McGraw-Hill.

Sulmasy, D. P., Lehmann, L. S., Levine, D. M. and Faden, R. R. (1994).

Patients' perceptions of the quality of informed consent for common medical procedures. *Journal of Clinical Ethics*, **5**, 189–194.

Sumerling, R. (1994). Therapeutic responsibility and the law. In *The Healing Bond: The Patient–Practitioner Relationship and Therapeutic Responsibility* (S. Budd and U. Sharma, eds), London: Routledge.

Swain, J. (1995). *The Use of Counselling Skills: A Guide for Therapists*. Oxford: Butterworth-Heinemann.

Thomasma, D. C. (1994). Telling the truth to patients: a clinical ethics exploration. *Cambridge Quarterly of Healthcare Ethics*, **3**, 375–382.

Thompson, I. E. (1979). The nature of confidentiality. *Journal of Medical Ethics*, **5**, 57–64.

Thompson, I. E. (1990). Ethics. In *Occupational Therapy in Mental Health: Principles, Skills and Practice* (J. Creek, ed.), Edinburgh: Churchill Livingstone.

Tobias, J. S. and Souhami, R. L. (1993). Fully informed consent can be needlessly cruel. *British Medical Journal*, **307**, 1199–1201.

Toon, P. D. (1993). After bioethics and towards virtue? *Journal of Medical Ethics*, **19**, 17–18.

Trowell, H. (1973). *The Unfinished Debate on Euthanasia*. London: SCM Press.

Tschudin, V. (1992). *Ethics in Nursing: The Caring Relationship*, 2nd edn. Oxford: Butterworth-Heinemann.

Tuohey, J. F. (1995). Moving from autonomy to responsibility in HIV-related healthcare. *Cambridge Quarterly of Healthcare Ethics*, **4**, 64–70.

Turnbull, H. R., Guess, D., Backus, L. H. *et al.* (1986). A model for analyzing the moral aspects of special education and behavioral interventions: the moral aspects of aversive procedures. In *Ethics of Dealing with Persons with Severe Handicaps: Toward a Research Agenda* (R. D. Dokecki and R. M. Zaner, eds), Baltimore: Paul H. Brookes Publishing.

UKCC (1993). United Kingdom Central Council for Nursing, Midwifery and Health Visiting. Advice to nurses on AIDS, and records. *Bulletin of Medical Ethics*, **91** (Sept), 8–11.

Veatch, R. M. (1973). Generalization of expertise: scientific expertise and value judgments. *Hastings Center Studies*, **1** (May), 29–40.

Veatch, R. M. (1981). *A Theory of Medical Ethics*. New York: Basic Books.

Veatch, R. M. (1988). Justice and the economics of terminal illness. *Hastings Center Report*, **18**, 34-40.

Venesy, B. A. (1994). A clinician's guide to decision making capacity and ethically sound medical decisions. *American Journal of Physical Medicine and Rehabilitation*, **73**, 219-226.

Vines, P. (1996). Informed consent: from paternal benevolence to trust mediated by truthfulness. *Australian Journal of Physiotherapy*, **42**, 245-246.

Walters, L. (1978). Ethical aspects of medical confidentiality. In *Contemporary Issues in Bioethics* (T. L. Beauchamp and L. Walters, eds), Encino: Dickenson Publishing .

Warnock, G. J. (1971). *The Object of Morality*. London: Methuen.

Waymack, M. H. (1991). Old age and the rationing of scarce health care resources. In *Aging and Ethics: Philosophical Problems in Gerontology* (N. S. Jecker, ed.), Totowa: Humana Press.

Wear, S. (1993). *Informed Consent: Patient Autonomy and Physician Beneficence within Clinical Medicine*. Dordrecht: Kluwer Academic Publishers.

Wilding, P. (1982). *Professional Power and Social Welfare*. London: Routledge. & Kegan Paul.

Williams, A. (1985). Economics of coronary artery bypass grafting. *British Medical Journal*, **281**, 326-329.

Williams, B. (1976). Utilitarianism and moral self-indulgence. In *Contemporary British Philosophy: Personal Statements - 4th Series* (H. D. Lewis, ed.), London: George Allen & Unwin.

Williamson, C. (1992). *Whose Standards? Consumer and Professional Standards in Health Care*. Buckingham: Open University Press.

Wright, C. (1973). Personal view. *British Medical Journal*, **4**, 45.

Index